PROFESSOR
PAUL LEE

Regeneration by Design

The science
of superhuman ageing

R^ethink

DISCLAIMER

This book is not intended as a substitute for professional
medical advice. It is not meant, nor should it be used, to
diagnose or treat any medical condition. Readers are advised
to consult a medical professional for specific diagnosis and
treatment, and before making any changes to their healthcare
regime or treatment. Neither the author nor the publisher will
be liable for any damages arising out of or in connection with
the use of this book.

Contents

Foreword

By Sharron Davies, MBE

Embarking on the journey of *Regeneration By Design* by Professor Paul YF Lee, I found myself not just reading a book, but engaging in a transformative experience that reshapes our understanding of health, vitality, and the potential to live our lives to the fullest, irrespective of age.

As someone who has navigated the highs of Olympic competition and the lows of physical wear to my joints, I have sought solutions that extend beyond the conventional. Professor Lee's approach to regenerative medicine, which I have had the privilege to experience first-hand, not only redefined my understanding of recovery and health but also offered a glimpse into the future of holistic wellbeing.

Regeneration By Design is not merely about ageing gracefully; it's a manifesto for revolutionising our approach to our bodies and our health. Professor Lee combines his expertise in orthopaedics, elite sports medicine and innovative engineering to help us unlock our regenerative superpowers. This book is a treasure trove of knowledge, blending physics, chemistry and biology to chart a course for enhanced musculoskeletal function and optimal health.

Through the Six Superhuman Steps, Professor Lee guides us to minimise disturbances that impair our body's natural healing capacity, urging us to rethink how we live, eat and move. His strategic use of AI and digital technology empowers us to take control of our health destiny, crafting a personalised blueprint for regeneration.

Regeneration By Design encapsulates this philosophy, providing practical tools and insights to navigate the complexities of modern healthcare and make informed decisions about our wellbeing. My journey so far has taught me that true strength lies in our capacity to regenerate and adapt.

This book is a call to action – to embrace a life of superhuman vitality through the power of science and innovation. Whether you are an athlete, a professional, or anyone in pursuit of peak health, *Regeneration By Design* offers a blueprint to thrive in a world where living well means embracing the science of regeneration.

Sharron Davies, MBE, Olympian, broadcaster and advocate for health and wellbeing

Foreword

by Professor Jonathan Whitehead

I was first introduced to Paul in late 2019 by a colleague who thought that we had overlapping research interests and complementary personalities.

On the former, they were correct! Having studied the biology of fat tissue and fat cells for over twenty years, I was fascinated to learn that Paul, along with other pioneers in the field, was using fat tissue isolated from a patient's abdomen to treat their osteoarthritic knees. Soon after talking with Paul, he arranged for me to watch him perform the procedure up close on two of his patients. His ability to put his patients at ease, whilst performing a series of steps to harvest and process the 'micro-fragmented adipose tissue' ready for injection into the affected knee, impressed me, particularly his unique style when fragmenting the adipose tissue – think of Tom Cruise 'flairing' in the film *Cocktail*. Subsequent rigorous analysis of the results of around fifty consecutive procedures showed that all had elicited positive outcomes, with the arthritis significantly improving in all cases. Whilst the molecular mechanisms underpinning these beneficial effects remain elusive it seems highly likely that a combination of Paul's four pillars, namely physics, chemistry, biology and time, all play a role.

Since then, Paul's energy, drive, enthusiasm and vision have remained a regular source of inspiration.

I feel many people would define Paul as a 'can-do' person. However, I think this would be selling him short and believe it is more appropriate to describe him as a 'will-do' person, the main question being how *soon* will he do it. This will-do approach is aligned with a healthy appetite to devour the research literature as well as other complementary resources to ensure he is at the cutting edge of the field of regeneration. One example of this is his collaboration with leading academics in the field of medical imaging and computer vision to develop Musculoskeletal Action Imaging technology, MAI-Motion. This integrates AI-driven 3D motion and 3D volumetric MRI analysis to provide more holistic insights that will aid in the diagnosis, management and rehabilitation of musculoskeletal issues. Paul's intention is to make the essence of this approach, suitably captured and distilled in the phrase 'Digital Kinematic Signature', accessible to most of us through the not-so-humble, but fairly ubiquitous, smartphone camera. Further evidence of Paul's unique will-do persona is his ability to attract colleagues, collaborators, patients and others who are outside his immediate field, to engage, provide input and contribute opinions.

Whilst Paul appears to have enjoyed a relatively classic clinical education, like many of us who have been around for more than a few years, he is happy to challenge and reinterpret dogma when presented with new evidence. Paul's recognition of Caplan's revised interpretation of his acclaimed work describing Mesenchymal Stem Cells to the less celebrated Medicinal Signalling Cells, highlights this. Paul's own insistence that there should be due consideration of the potential negative impact of steroid injections (on the balance between regeneration and degeneration) to treat an arthritic joint before administering such provides further evidence of his ability to reflect on the status quo and act appropriately.

Finally, returning to the latter part of my opening statement. For the attributes mentioned above, I can conclude that Paul and I do indeed have complementary traits and personalities. And it is because of these attributes that he is recognised and held in such high esteem by all those who interact with him, whether they be patients, colleagues or collaborators.

This book, *Regeneration By Design*, provides a unique overview of the current state-of-the-art of regeneration based on the experience and perspective of Professor Paul Lee, one of the leaders in the field of musculoskeletal and regenerative medicine. His vision, communicated in this book, is to help us all move a little closer to our superhuman selves.

Jonathan Whitehead, Professor of Biomedical Biochemistry, University of Lincoln

Introduction

Superpowers represent a fantasy we all have, surely. What would it mean to be 'superhuman'? Some of us would choose to fly, others might pick invisibility or Hulk-like strength or the ability to time travel. If we are honest, however, living forever would surely top the list. Eternal youth, eternal life and eternal love – we may deny it but these are the things that we all desire. Yet, we must be careful what we wish for. Does living for longer, let alone forever, always mean living better? The evidence, when it comes to our mobility and physical health, suggests otherwise.

More of us are increasingly living with varying degrees of pain thanks to an epidemic of bone, joint and muscle damage. We are not, as a general population, ageing particularly well. Worryingly, it seems we have come to accept aches and pains as we advance in years. As a champion of regenerative medicine, I find this attitude incredibly frustrating and have written this book to challenge it with an alternative, positive outlook. There is nothing inevitable about discomfort as we get older. We can, and should, fight back. Consider this book a rallying cry for superhumans to assemble and resist musculoskeletal decline. To help, it turns out we do not need special powers to enjoy a healthy life as we get older. We can make it happen through design.

In *Regeneration By Design,* I propose a new philosophy of regenerative medicine and demonstrate how the sciences – physics, chemistry and biology – help us fight the effects of getting on in years. I share the latest innovations in musculoskeletal care and provide life lessons that will help you take better care of your muscles, bones and joints. As the saying goes, 'Failure to plan is planning to fail'. Reading this book will put your destiny back into your hands by giving you a set of principles you can use to plan how you age. As I do this, you won't find me recommending the shortcuts or 'bio-hacks' that gain attention in the press and social media. They might well be helpful and, after all, we share a goal – the promotion of health. My approach is, however, more considered and medically proven.

When I am not writing books, my day-to-day work is as an orthopaedic surgeon. Despite enjoying my job a great deal, my starting point, as I first put pen to paper, was an assumption that readers would prefer *not* to go under my scalpel. Despite being relatively routine these days, treating damaged joints by removing them and inserting manmade metal and plastic apparatuses in their place is always a relatively serious operation that comes with inherent risks. It probably counts as a course of action that we should avoid if we possibly can.

My preference, by far, is helping patients mature in years without surgery and so I am an enthusiastic supporter of protecting bones, joints and muscles before even minor problems occur. Should damage happen, it is surely better to instigate a repair of the affected joint than rush to replace it. Such thinking has driven my career from the very beginning. Since my early days at medical school, I have combined my interest in scrubbing up and getting to grips with patients' issues in the operating theatre with developing a broader understanding of musculoskeletal health through laboratory research. Thanks to this, over the years, I have had a front-row seat during many of regenerative medicine's most exciting developments.

My qualifications and experience have found a natural home in sports science. Besides my medical degree, I have an MSc in Sports Medicine alongside surgical fellowships in regenerative medicine and a PhD in Medical Cell Engineering. I have spent a fair proportion of my time with the nearest thing we have to real superhumans and investigating musculoskeletal issues for a range of elite athletes, including world-renowned footballers, international rugby players, Olympic swimmers and world-class marathon runners.

How does this help you? The answer is, today, every single aspect of an elite sportsperson's physiology is scientifically measured. You don't have to follow sports in any detail to imagine the huge amounts of time and effort spent in finding even the smallest of competitive advantages. Our understanding of how damage and regeneration work within sportspeople is incredibly advanced as a result.

Sadly, many of the lessons we have learned through sports science seem to be forgotten or ignored by doctors when faced with Joe Public. Medicine for the general population and sports medicine are somewhat at arm's length from each other. This seems a particularly unhelpful state of affairs. There are, after all, no reasons why the same principles that lie behind returning an injured Premiership footballer to the team or keeping a world-class runner on the road, can't help us all stay mobile. All of us have the potential to be superhuman, after all.

Our later years can be a beautiful stage of life. We should all, for example, feel reassured by fine wine. Connoisseurs know that good bottles improve over the years. They don't, however, leave this improvement to chance. There are rules to storing wine correctly, including temperature, humidity and light levels. The kitchen cupboard will certainly not do. It is the same with any human achievement. The world's great architecture is another illustration. It is ridiculous to think the Empire State Building, for example, happened by chance. You wouldn't ever conceive of building a skyscraper without doing a bit of studying, planning and designing, would you? Now, imagine what spending time, care and attention on designing our lives around a fit and active future could achieve. This is why I want to redefine regenerative medicine and broaden the population it is applied to. Wouldn't it be amazing if our musculoskeletal health didn't feel as though it were in the lap of the gods? If we could design it, wouldn't we feel superhuman?

Those looking for a quick fix for their general health or a basic self-help book may be slightly disappointed by *Regeneration By Design*. I shall not be simply telling you to monitor your weight, eat healthily or do more exercise (although we should all be doing those things). Instead, the book is a crystallisation of all I have learned throughout my career, including clinical exchanges with superhuman sportspeople. I have aimed to translate the latest in regenerative medicine to be useful in your everyday life – not just today, but for many years to come. As the saying goes, 'Give a person a fish and you feed him for a day. Teach a person to fish and you feed him for a lifetime'.

I have written this book for everyone. It is never too early or too late to start applying *Regeneration By Design*'s principles. Alongside theory, I have included practical steps you can take at any age to improve your bone, joint and muscular health. Even if you just adopt a small selection of the action points that I propose, you will feel more in control. As I do this, it is important to note that regeneration by design should not start from guilt or embarrassment. I have seen many people, motivated by a sense of shame, compensate for a sedentary youth by overexerting themselves in middle age. Rushing back to the squash court to make amends for years of inactivity is not a route to superhuman status. It is more likely to lead to ruptured tendons, torn ligaments and worse. Anything done in haste is best avoided. My suggestions are mercifully less dramatic and based on making incremental changes to your routine. In this book, for example, you will learn that even the simple act of smiling releases endorphins that support our powers of regeneration. Getting a good night's sleep helps too. It is truly the little things that matter.

Regeneration is a matter of maintaining the finest of balances. Homeostasis is a key concept to understand what this means. The term describes the body's natural ability to maintain a steady internal environment despite changes in external conditions. Healthy joints continually swing between degeneration and regeneration in a continual search for stability. The processes involved are complex and systemic, meaning traditional interventions such as surgery seem overly simple and mechanistic. Replacing a hip in isolation may not help because there is always the surrounding muscle and tendon to consider, for example. It doesn't stop there. What about the legs, trunk and spine? Even the performance of our shoulders and necks can be affected by how we walk. There is an interconnection of movement within our body. The way that the joints interact with each other and the movement pattern of the human body has a huge influence on the way that we live. This interaction is difficult to define, but I call it our 'Digital Kinematic Signature' as we all have our own. It's not just about velocity and force. The smoothness of movement, control and symmetry all play a part in our unique signatures.

Electrical signals, chemical instructions and biological conditions all add to the picture too. This means finding a balance means considering everything from our DNA to our vitamin intake and everything in between. The list goes on and on, so it pays to always look at the big picture. This is why, as well as framing the problem of today's regenerative medicine and proposing improvements, I have included chapters on physics, chemistry and biology in *Regeneration By Design*. There is, however, no need to worry if you're a general reader. These chapters are designed to prompt new thinking rather than teach as a science textbook might. You can relax, although I have written textbooks on the subject, I have no desire to take you back to school here.

The future of regenerative medicine is, I believe, an incredibly exciting one. It is an area I champion evangelically to such an extent that I'm known as 'The Regeneration Man' in certain circles. Today, science gives us the potential to make a real difference in how, and when, we experience getting older. Success, however, is dependent on moving away from mechanistic interventions when surgeons take a narrow view of fixing joints. Having learned so much about the benefits of a broader, more systemic approach through treating the superhumans of the track and field, it is surely time to think and act differently.

To reiterate my opening position, I cannot promise you actual superpowers as some authors or 'biohackers' on the fringes of science seem to. I do, however, want you to learn some regenerative principles and design your life based on current, proven regenerative medicine. As a little bonus for readers, I have included some further reading in the form of previously published articles covering specific musculoskeletal, regeneration and artificial intelligence issues. This will, I trust, help you face the future like a superhuman and keep you well away from my operating table.

As a final introductory note, this book isn't an endeavour I can claim sole credit for. It builds on the excellent work of a huge number of other scientists and engineers. As a scientist and engineer myself, it is only appropriate for me to share one of my favourite quotes from Sir Isaac Newton: 'If I see further, it is because I am standing on the shoulders of giants.'[1]

ONE

An Overview Of Regenerative Medicine

Today, it is widely acknowledged that far too many of us experience muscle pain and joint degeneration as we get older. Despite a huge explosion in the amount of information available today on health and well-being, there is little agreement on what we ought to do about it. There are many health gurus, hackers and influencers who are more than happy to talk about running, losing fat and eating less carbs. Their advice and perspectives are all taken from the cardiovascular sections of medical textbooks: burn energy, raise your heartbeat and stay healthy. There is, by comparison, very little talk of our musculoskeletal health.

We collectively seem to have decided that our bone and joint health is something we can put off worrying about until later. Maybe because our movement has always been present in our lives, we take it for granted. This is human nature, of course. We are all busy doing other things in our lives and so we've become adept at denial and procrastination. We will think about the health of our joints in the future; tomorrow, next week, in a few years and so on. It never seems to be today, this minute or now. We tend to only consult our doctors and seek help when our symptoms have become intolerable. We typically only ask for help once we are in too much pain to cope and our ability to enjoy life is being compromised. We rarely, if ever, consider seeking help before it is too late.

As a result, in its present form, regenerative medicine feels like it is a reactive and underperforming science. At its worst, it is not recognised at all. I have written *Regeneration By Design* to view the subject through fresh eyes and inspire readers to act with a renewed sense of urgency. I believe regenerative medicine can, and should, make a significant impact on our general health. It can help guide us and identify issues that will steer us towards superhuman status immediately rather than, as we tend to do, wait until we have a problem before acting.

Back pain epidemic

As an example of the problems associated with musculoskeletal procrastination, through my work I see many office workers of a certain age being forced to adapt their working patterns because of chronic back pain. They might go as far as standing at modified desks rather than adopting the traditional sitting and typing setup. Frustratingly, by the time I become aware of them, they are doing this to alleviate existing back pain symptoms. They have, tragically, gone way past the point where preventative measures would make a difference. They have acted too late to stop damage to the back from occurring in the first place.

Back pain is a good place to start a discussion of the current problematic state of regenerative medicine because, inarguably, it is the most widespread musculoskeletal problem the world faces today. Discussing back pain in the context of regenerative medicine is akin to addressing the mammoth in the room. By 2050, the number of people suffering from lower back pain globally is expected to reach nearly a billion – that's comparable to the entire population of India.

In the UK, back pain affects six out of every ten people, roughly the same proportion of those who own a car. The economic impact of back pain in the UK is staggering, costing the economy up to £10.7 billion in lost work time every year. That's the same cost as running the London Underground for a year. The NHS spends the equivalent of the 2012 London Olympic budget (£4.76 billion) every year on back pain. Shockingly, nearly a third of all NHS GP appointments revolve around musculoskeletal issues. In 2023, that meant over 300,000 people looked for help every day.[2]

Understanding the statistics on back pain becomes even more astonishing when we consider that required preventive measures are simpler than the routine maintenance of a car. Imagine the twenty-five intervertebral discs in your spine as sponges, each composed of 95% water. Just as a sponge dries out and becomes brittle without water, a lack of hydration leads to the degeneration of these discs. This deterioration can happen at a rate as alarming as 1% per year, meaning by the age of fifty, you could lose nearly half the cartilage in these vital spinal cushions. Without proper maintenance – in this case, the recommended 6–8 cups of fluid daily – the vertebrae in your spine could end up grinding against each other and causing pain. This is comparable to a car's metal parts clashing due to worn-out tyres. Adequate hydration can keep backs healthy much like well-inflated car tyres prevent a bumpy ride.

This is just one example of the impact that proactive regenerative medicine can have. Later in the book, we will discuss the endorphins you get simply by smiling. There really is no excuse for failing to look after ourselves.

Part of the problem is we often forget that degenerative processes occur throughout our bodies naturally. All our joints, bones and muscles decay. It is part of our cellular makeup. It is, in fact, part of being alive. What matters is that we design regenerative steps in response.

Regeneration and degeneration

I am far too much of an optimist to write a book entirely about death, but I fear we must discuss it briefly to introduce the basic ideas and concepts surrounding the ageing process. To understand death and our inevitable journey towards it, we must discuss the continual battle between regeneration and degeneration going on in our bodies.

In fact, we can actually define death as the total loss of our bodies' ability to regenerate. Death, proven science tells us, is the end of a continuous biochemical battle. Our demise marks degeneration's final victory in the one contest we can never win. I've often thought the aphorism about the inevitability of death and taxes is inaccurate. Creative accountants may be able to help with tax planning. There is no arguing with the first part, though. Once life is over, there's no coming back. Whether wealthy or impoverished, a monarch or a mendicant, extraordinarily ambitious or simply content with the ordinary, the inexorable march of the Grim Reaper spares none, uniting us all in the common destiny of life's end.

Aware that the subject drives every aspect of our lives, students of molecular biology have, over the years, turned their attention to death too. We now know more about the processes that lead to our final departures than ever. For example, we have discovered that the vast majority of our cells are actively programmed to die. After a certain amount of time, determined by our DNA, programmed cell death kicks in through a process called apoptosis and healthy cells begin to die off. It is a perfectly natural process; a terminal mechanism that is part of our makeup and forms the circle of life from the moment we are born.

Cells, of course, can also be killed by trauma and disease. If you drive your car into a tree, the resulting accident will prove fatal if too many of your cells are killed as a result. If you develop infections or disease then the process is the same, except it happens over a much longer, drawn-out and distressing period. Known as necrosis, cells dying because of external factors in this way help us shuffle off the mortal coil at various speeds and with varying degrees of success.

A third set of cells plays a role in our expiration. In a process we don't yet fully understand, healthy cells can simply forget the apoptosis process. This doesn't count as necrosis because it's not caused by anything external. Rather than die as programmed, this third class of cells is seized by a need to live and reproduce. Those that do, mutate and replicate uncontrollably at a huge cost to their hosts. Left unchecked, they prove fatal. We call these cells cancerous.

It is not all doom and gloom. Some cells, such as those in our muscles, blood, skin, hair, nails, digestive tracts, reproductive systems and more, can, and do, replicate themselves. This is through a simple process of natural cell division and self-cloning known as mitosis. Thanks to mitosis, a single human cell can divide into two genetically identical daughter cells. New cells created in this way are crucial for the growth and repair that takes place in our bodies and keep us all cycling through life, death and rebirth. It is a very important process in regenerative medicine.

Sadly, we all ultimately depart because cells undergoing mitosis in our bodies are always outnumbered by other cells; those falling foul of apoptosis, those dying through necrotic external influences and, if we're unlucky, those turning into cancer.

Even healthy cells can't go on forever. The DNA sequences and proteins required to multiply cells, known as telomeres, get shorter and shorter with each cell division. When they get too short, cells lose the ability to divide naturally. Overall, we are never entirely or exactly balanced. Despite our best efforts, cellular biology means the scales always ultimately favour degeneration and we are continually tipped downwards on a mortal trajectory to the end. I am aware this is a slightly depressing view of the human condition. *Regeneration By Design* is certainly not intended to be depressing, so I shan't dwell on death any longer. Suffice to say it is useful to think of our healthy bodies as home to twin processes; those which constantly renew, regenerate and heal and those which see healthy cells die an inevitable natural death. When things are going well, these two competing processes keep everything stable.

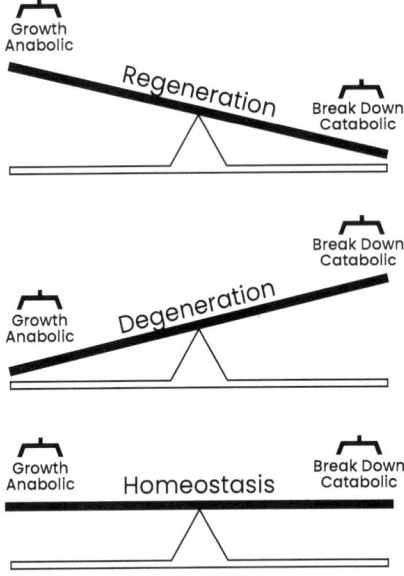

Regeneration versus degeneration and homeostasis

A healthy body regulates itself despite external influences. Various feedback mechanisms, controlled by physics, chemistry and biology, work together to maintain a natural state of equilibrium known as homeostasis, albeit with degeneration always having the upper hand. When it comes to your joints, bones and muscles, I intend to share ways to keep this healthy balance. Where degeneration and damage happen, we can apply regenerative methods and treatments to compensate. This is key to staying in control and designing how we respond to more years on the clock.

Before leaving this section, however, I am aware that there are those on the fringes of science that, at the time of writing, are exploring radical, and notably, expensive methodologies to interrupt or sidestep molecular and cellular biology. In my view, they are on a fool's errand. Rather than challenge unstoppable forces, living to a ripe old age will always be the result of working with nature rather than against it. My position is that we will never be able to cheat degeneration and death. We can, however, certainly make decisions that may delay the inevitable and help us age well. *The secret is to understand the science behind our present and plan for the future.* Regeneration by design is always going to be preferable to leaving your well-being to chance.

Leaving regeneration to chance

It might be helpful to steer away from superhumans briefly to talk about supercars. In purchasing one, most would naturally gravitate towards renowned manufacturers like Lamborghini or Ferrari, known for their expertise, prestige, history and advanced scientific facilities. There are cheaper ways to achieve the same result though. Kit cars exist. You can invest in body and engine modifications that mimic supercar effects. These are, however, never quite the same, are they? It is the same with superhumans. Shortcuts and quick modifications cannot compete with tried and trusted engineering. This is why I always turn to established science and design.

We can use our car analogy to develop this idea further. Imagine deciding to buy a classic Porsche 959 or Ferrari Testarossa and, rather than ask for a finished vehicle, asking for all its constituent parts to be delivered and simply left, unboxed, on your garage floor. You can look at the thousands of parts in hope for days, months or even years, but very little is going to happen if you do not act. Perhaps, then, after a long time just looking, you decide to do just that. Your plan? To simply throw every single one of your supercar components up into the air to see if they might land in exactly the right places to form the finished car. Technically, this might actually work. One day could, indeed, be an incredibly lucky day and your trillion-to-one gamble might pay off. Each component might land in exactly the right place at the right time. It would inarguably count as a never-to-be-repeated, truly miraculous outcome of truly cosmic proportions, but it could happen.

In the real world, of course, we know the above example is patently ridiculous. A beautifully engineered sports car could never be the result of random activity. A pile of components could never actually just fall into place. We know a Porsche 959 or Ferrari Testarossa is the result of hundreds, if not thousands, of hours of work. Highly complex and innovative production lines and intricate, skilled workmanship are involved in their creation. There is the brainpower of hundreds of skilled designers, engineers and technicians to consider too. It is surely fair to say there is nothing remotely random about a Porsche or a Ferrari.

Why am I sharing this with you? Well, it was a favourite analogy of my mentor, Professor James Richardson of Robert Jones and Agnes Hunt Orthopaedic Hospital. He would use it to describe the job of regenerating cartilage in a knee joint, but it applies to all musculoskeletal interventions. Simply implanting the 'ingredients' and hoping for a successful outcome rarely leads to the desired outcome.

Professor Richardson, who knew more than most that a knee joint is every bit as complicated as a sports car, was not a fan of leaving things to chance. He would urge doctors and patients alike to apply sound scientific and engineering principles to fix problems. It is a lesson I have applied throughout my career and is, in fact, a major inspiration behind this book. The amount of design, thought, effort, time and resources you put into regeneration will shape the results.

I ought to add a note about statistics. Whenever you discuss these matters, you will find unhelpful outliers who claim to have beaten the odds without any effort at all. They will tell you of a relative or friend (it is rarely themselves, of course) who has beaten the odds by chance. The friend will have drunk red wine every day of their lives and lived to the age of 103.

They might also have smoked five packs of cigarettes a day and missed out on lung cancer. Another friend might have played rugby since they were a child and not had a single ache or pain. Such stories might make you question the evidence.

The numbers don't lie, though. According to Cancer UK, the lung cancer risk is around twenty-six times higher in men who smoke compared to those who never started and, on average,[3] almost fifty injuries take place for every 1000 hours of play in men's senior amateur rugby union according to a 2018 research paper.[4] The reason we hear from outliers is because they feel they have beaten the system. Winning the lottery in life is worthy of celebrating. Those who suffer the consequences of their actions in line with statistical, rather than anecdotal, evidence tend to keep quiet about it. There is little point in listening to people who claim to have beaten the ageing odds through luck, in any case. There is no useful information to be gained from outcomes that have happened by chance. Useful information comes from patients who have beaten the odds by making sound, evidence-based choices. The good news is I have written *Regeneration By Design* with this very much in mind.

Waiting too long to start

When should you start thinking about your regenerative health? The questions I am asked more than any other in my clinical practice are all variations of a theme: when. When should I start my treatment? When should I have my operation? When should I get back to work? When can I train again? When will I be able to run again? When will I be fit again? I've dedicated a whole chapter to the context of time later in the book but the universal truth is the sooner you get help, the quicker any treatment will be, the sooner your problem can be fixed and the faster you can be back at your best.

So, when I'm asked about when to start, my answer is always now. You may have picked up this book because you have felt a twinge in your lower back or your left knee is starting to feel sore when you run. Do something about that today. Seek professional help and prevent further damage. If you haven't any symptoms, what then? What if you're feeling fine and healthy? Should you still start thinking about regenerative medicine? Again, I'd say yes. There is no time like the present to start designing your future.

I should, perhaps, interject here with a small note of caution. There's no need to do anything in haste. For many of us, change can be challenging. Many self-styled gurus and self-help writers of the kind you often see in the US talk about making changes in your life without hesitation. They sell the idea that success is the result of immediate action. For them, success happens when you make big, profound and lasting changes to your life. To truly capture all our psychological drive and enthusiasm, any change in direction, in their opinion, needs to be quick and radical. Habits need to be broken and rebuilt. Our routines and rituals need to be renewed and refreshed. In other words, 'Fortune favours the brave,' or to borrow from one of the world's favourite brands, 'Just Do It.'

This may be effective in business, relationships and many other areas of life. Infectious, motivational messages do, to be fair, have a good track record of success and certainly sell a lot of books. I am, however, less convinced by this approach when it comes to becoming superhuman. I talked about the risk of injury from over-committing to a return to squash in middle age in the book's introduction. I am aware this doesn't sound overly dramatic or exciting, and it's far from your typical superhuman origin story, but I'm not entirely sure that regenerative medicine ought to feel radical at all. To borrow from *Aesop's Fables*, regeneration by design might be a case of the slow and steady tortoise winning out in the end.

To help illustrate my point further, think of driving the Porsche or Ferrari you imagined earlier in the chapter. Picture spotting something ahead of you on the road blocking your way. You might be tempted to slam on the brakes and pull a handbrake turn as if you are a stuntman taking part in a superhero movie car chase. Why not? What is your imagination for if you can't have a little bit of fun? In the real world, however, you would want to react calmly, safely and responsibly behind the wheel. This may not be as sexy or entertaining, but it does keep everyone safe.

Why don't we park the sports car analogy briefly and try something bigger, on the ocean waves perhaps? Captains of the latest ultra-large oil tankers that cross the Pacific spend every moment on deck planning far ahead. They routinely turn off the engines of their huge vessels up to 25 kilometres out of port. This is the distance they need to slow down and come to a stop at the right spot. The *RMS Titanic*, God rest her, spotted the iceberg 370 miles off the coast of Newfoundland well enough, but had too much momentum to turn sufficiently to avoid it. In general, fast cars and big ships are not good at change. You don't have to have studied the human condition in much depth to realise that, despite encouragement, people are generally not very good at it either. This is especially true when it comes to getting older. I often ask my patients to change habits they have developed over their entire lifetimes so to expect massive action and immediate results is perhaps asking a little too much.

To my mind, regenerative medicine, the science of getting older like a superhuman, is based on the sensible notion that we should avoid as many icebergs and bumps in the road as possible. Our bodies will inevitably throw degenerative problems at us. And we need to plan for those we can't avoid. How can we respond to this challenge? There are people we can look to as examples of success. If we take showbusiness, for example, it is no accident that Tom Cruise looks forever young. Cruise is still performing stunts in his sixties and, as demonstrated by making a *Top Gun* sequel twenty-five years after the original, is still a box office draw. In the UK, David Beckham is also looking ridiculously good for his age, despite giving up playing over a decade ago. Both, it is clear, have invested considerable resources in their health, fitness and well-being. We can also think of celebrities who look older than their years. It is perhaps impolite to name them, but you can tell that they have committed to rock and roll lifestyles rather than planned for future fitness.

It will be interesting to see how today's crop of Premiership footballers age. They are under huge pressure to perform and win games, so that is where their focus lies. They have little time to think about regeneration as they play. It only becomes an issue when they have an injury, which is usually a little too late. To help square this circle, some of today's top sports stars and celebrities are considering a process labelled 'biobanking'. This is a way of preparing for later regenerative needs by storing huge amounts of biological data and keeping a record of their younger selves to aid their future older selves. It's an exciting approach that might one day work for everyone, so I discuss it in some detail later in the book.

Although it's exciting to ponder the lives of the rich and famous, this book is much more about more mundane, small, straightforward incremental changes designed to help you better navigate the route to superhuman status. I will ask you to think about how you sit, stand and move around, but you can relax. I am not expecting anyone to take up marathon running or tackle the Tour de France as a result of anything they read here – unless they want to, of course. I am more in the business of sharing tips and ideas for relatively minor adjustments. I'll also share the physics, chemistry and biology behind the tips, because a little scientific understanding makes it easier to change your habits.

Summary

All in all, if you're worried about the advancing years and their impact on your joints and mobility, you've made a great start by reading the first chapter of the book. I hope it has set the scene for what is to follow. There's no right time to start thinking about regeneration, but the longer you leave it, the harder making the changes I am suggesting will become. The risk of degenerative damage and related pain only increases with time. It is no exaggeration to say everyone I see in pain at my orthopaedic clinics wishes they had started thinking about their musculoskeletal health earlier. Why not act like a superhuman and start right now?

TWO

A New Philosophy

Having set the scene, I now feel more confident introducing you to my superhuman approach to regenerative medicine. Unlike the fantasy of the movies, it centres on tackling the problem of regeneration scientifically, systematically and by design.

If we take a very high-level view, regeneration is no different from any other problem humanity has faced. History has taught us that the best way to attack such problems is through science and engineering. As a species, we have achieved great things through the robust application of tried-and-tested design methodologies. We have, for example, eradicated smallpox and beaten Covid-19. We have mapped the human genome, found the Higgs boson particle, sent men to the Moon and put a telescope in orbit to photograph galaxies 13.6 billion light-years from Earth. I could go on. The list is endless. We have engineers to thank for all these great leaps forward and I discuss their influence in more depth in the next chapter.

Here, I'll share where my *Regeneration By Design* philosophy comes from and how it will help you get the most out of what follows. I champion the belief that the key to improving regenerative health can be found using scientific disciplines and engineering principles. Time is also very important to consider, because with time, things change. It is also a currency we all have in common. Knowing when to intervene, as well as how to, is incredibly important in my line of work.

Before getting into detail, it is probably worth taking time to discuss how my thinking developed. It started with my experience treating elite sportspeople, the 'superhumans', and noting that lessons hadn't necessarily been applied to general medicine. This is, at least in part, because solving complex problems is difficult and overcoming established medical dogma is challenging.

Lessons from sports science

Based on sound scientific principles and evidence, we know it is possible to design technological systems that make our lives easier. We use them in the form of a myriad of machines and devices every day. Biological systems, such as those we see in nature and, ultimately, within ourselves, prove more challenging to figure out because they are much more complex. However, we have made massive strides in understanding how our bodies work and how to keep them in top condition in recent years. The new ideas, excellent research and significant innovations that have led me to coin the term 'superhumans' have inarguably come from the elite sports field. Talented sports scientists have studied the physics of our motions, the chemistry of nutrition and the biology of our life support processes in the constant hunt for competitive advantage. As a result, they have become a key source of innovation.

As general medical professionals, we can use information gained from sports stars in the same way the motor industry has long used Formula One's racing discoveries. A well-resourced Formula One team continually innovates and its members become experts in the systems and processes required to win races: accelerating, braking, changing gear, steering and overtaking. We can see this knowledge filter down to improve the performance of road cars available on the general market. Sport is your best bet for equivalent innovations in and around the human body for the same reasons. A Premier League football team is motivated by the need to win to understand the quickest way to repair a strained muscle, broken ankle or torn ligament, for example. Elite sports teams, more than any other organisations, can spend time, energy and money finding the most effective ways to get players off the injury bench and back in the fray. Money is very important. In the UK, we generally do not like to talk about it when it comes to our healthcare, but we do need to acknowledge that money and advances in technology go hand in hand. Without money, we would not have made many of the steps forward we celebrate today: MRI scans, motion tracking, genetic studies and so on. All these things cost money – and who has money? We are back to the world's elite sportspeople, their teams and supporting organisations.

I see my task as bringing twin stories together: elite sports and, for want of a better phrase, everyday medicine. Importantly, this doesn't mean I'm going to suggest you behave like a world record holder or an Olympic medallist. I shall not be recommending a training package, routine or regime for you. In fact, I am not interested in designing anything in your life at all. I won't tell you that you need to do twenty-five press-ups each morning, drink five litres of orange juice or cycle rather than drive to work. It is not going to be like that. You will have to design things for yourself. If the dieting industry tells us one thing, it is that 'life-changing' programmes that promise formulaic results don't always work. What I want to do, instead, is more subtle and nuanced. I want to give you information that adjusts the paradigms you live by. I want you to rethink how you view your body based on the principles I share with you.

These principles look at health as a way of correcting your body's balance more towards regeneration than degeneration. They have a deeper purpose than delivering single interventions and quick fixes. I intend to set you on a regenerative journey that will affect your life from today and for years to come.

In the chapters that follow, we will look at four pillars of regenerative medicine:

- Physics

- Chemistry

- Biology

- The context of time

The overriding message at the heart of *Regeneration By Design* is that most of us put insufficient thought into the above areas when we think of our bodies and ageing. If we don't plan our response to getting older, we are going to fail. If we don't design it, we won't be successful.

Complex problems

You may know that some species of lizards and some invertebrates have the natural ability to regenerate limbs after an attack by a predator. It is a feature of the natural world much beloved by TV documentaries and biology teachers, after all. We experience our own bodies naturally healing every day too. Most of us have scars from minor incidents that have occurred over the years. We can see regeneration is an innate, if imperfect, process. On the face of it, it is also quite a simple one. So much so, that beyond major trauma and illness, we rarely have to consciously think about it. If regeneration was simple, however, we would have learned exactly how it worked and replicated it by now and fighting ageing would be easy. The fact that it is not is a clear indication that regeneration is, in actuality, a complex and challenging subject.

Putting medicine aside for a moment, much thought has gone into how we, as human beings, approach problem-solving. Knowledge management and complex science researcher, David John Snowden has categorised the ways we perceive problems into four categories that are worth exploring:

1. Simple (or clear)

2. Complicated

3. Complex

4. Chaotic

It is worth running through them with reference to regeneration to frame the discussion and provide a bit of context to my thinking.[5]

'Simple problems' are generally well-defined. They have one input or cause and a single unambiguous solution. It might not feel like it, but building a flat-pack piece of furniture by following the instructions is a simple problem. At a stretch, in the world of medicine, you could describe fixing a fracture as a simple problem. Bind the bones together and let them heal. Does replacing a whole hip joint to ease the pain of arthritis count as simple, though? Despite the view held by some orthopaedic surgeons, I fear not. The number of variables involved in any surgery makes it complex.

In his second problem category, Snowden describes 'complicated problems' as similar to simple problems, but with the added complication of 'known unknown' factors between cause and solution. Following a map to drive between Leeds and London, for example, has one input (the journey) and one output (arrival). There are, however, a myriad of unexpected things that could happen on the way to complicate matters.

To give a very specific example, a warning light could begin to flash on your car dashboard as you drive to London (or anywhere, for that matter). This would count as a complicated problem. In most cars, you can read what the warning light means in the manual and make a judgement call about what needs to happen next, how and when. This is a complicated, but not hugely difficult, task because input and output are defined. It's the bit in the middle that contains variables.

The third of Snowden's categories is 'complex problems'. Here, complexity describes circumstances that could have multiple causes and multiple outcomes. The complexity is also compounded by 'unknown unknowns' in between. Imagine a machine that replicates fruit. Put in an apple and you get another apple. What could be simpler? Imagine it goes haywire and the outcomes become unpredictable. Put in an apple and you might get a banana. Put in a banana and you might get a teaspoon. Because the relationship between input and output has been broken, life has suddenly become more complex.

To illustrate this with a more concrete real-life example, let's go back to our problematic car journey. What if a warning light tells you something is wrong, but not what? There are many ways to attempt to solve the problem. You could research your warning light online, try and find a manual to refer to, take your car back to the manufacturer for help or visit multiple garages. With limited information, however, there is no guarantee anyone will find an answer. You may have to resort to trial and error. Yet, the warning light still comes on. At least some days. Some days it doesn't. This might appear to be related to the weather. Coldness or rain, perhaps. Could it be the route you're driving? The speed you are travelling at? The amount of braking you do? It is easy to see why the problem, with its myriad of variables, is described as complex.

How do we solve such complex problems, though? In reality, it is often the case that we don't bother trying. We simply ignore them. If it is simply a warning light, we will cope. If it is simply a twinge of back pain, we will make excuses for it and having done our own, sometimes unconscious, cost-benefit and risk calculations, decide that the best course of action, everything considered, is inaction.

We make this mistake because complex problems are, by definition, hard to solve. However, my experience of regenerative medicine is that they are not impossible. We make successful diagnoses every day. Treatments work. Patients get back on track. We can do this because, even in the face of complexity, we can turn to proven principles. Science, engineering and design methods won't fail us if we put the effort in.

The fourth of Snowden's categories is 'chaotic problems'. In this case, imagine driving your car into a wall and trying to fix it while everything is flying in all directions. If we are in the middle of a chaotic problem, we rarely react rationally. In medical terms, this could describe a major trauma where simple survival is the desired outcome.

Solutions through the lens of musculoskeletal regenerative medicine

Simple (Clear) – streamlining basic healing principles

Starting with the basics, we tackle simple health issues by embracing our body's natural ability to heal; similar to how it deals with minor cuts. We enhance this process by focusing on the essentials: good nutrition, staying active and proper care. These simple actions support our body's built-in repair system, promoting health and recovery in the most natural way.

Complicated – engineering precision solutions

When we face complicated health challenges, it's like navigating a tricky path that requires specialised knowledge and tools. In these cases, we apply advanced treatments, like stem cell therapy or custom rehabilitation programmes, designed specifically for an individual's unique health puzzle. This approach allows us to address these challenges with precision, offering a clear path to recovery.

Complex Problems – embracing systemic thinking

For complex issues, where unpredictability is the norm, we adopt a broader, more integrated strategy. This involves looking at the big picture and considering all factors that influence health. By incorporating advanced technologies like AI and machine learning, we can apply a wide array of regenerative treatments effectively, tailoring our approach to meet the nuanced needs of each individual.

Chaotic – navigating through innovation

In chaotic situations, characterised by severe unpredictability, the focus shifts to rapid, innovative solutions. These moments require us to be at the forefront of regenerative medicine, using the latest research and technology to navigate through the uncertainty and find new ways to heal and recover.

Applying it to musculoskeletal health

From simple to chaotic, regenerative medicine offers a range of solutions for musculoskeletal issues. For instance, fixing a broken bone is straightforward: aligning it properly and allowing it to heal. A more complicated scenario, like revising a knee replacement, involves removing old components and installing advanced ones. Treating cartilage damage in arthritis patients, a 'complex' problem, requires innovative regenerative strategies. And dealing with an acute infection, a 'chaotic' problem, demands quick, effective action to manage the crisis.

Replacing a damaged hip or painful knee may be complicated, but to an orthopaedic surgeon it is a relatively straightforward piece of problem-solving. Take out the worn bone and replace it with something new. Preventing the bone damage happening in the first place is, however, more like our car with an unidentifiable warning light. Thousands of variables might be at play, including the way we move, how much we are hydrated, our weight, our hobbies, our DNA, our choice of footwear, our heart health, a diabetes diagnosis, low blood pressure and so on. The list is extremely long. It is also individual to you. As a result, problem-solving becomes a complex issue and finding answers takes a new way of thinking guided by principles.

Strategies for addressing challenges in regenerative medicine: The regenerative approach

Category	Strategy	Key Actions	Outcome Focus
Simple (Clear)	Streamline basic principles	• Proper nutrition • Regular exercise • Routine care	Promote natural regeneration
Complicated	Engineer precision solutions	• Specialised knowledge • Advanced therapies • Personalised plans	Tailor treatments to individual needs
Complex Problems	Embrace systemic thinking	• Holistic assessment • AI integration • Adaptive solutions	Develop innovative solutions based on regenerative principles
Chaotic	Navigate through innovation	• Rapid response • Leverage research • Pioneer new pathways	Address emergencies and pioneer treatment advancements

Logic versus dogma

Change in the medical profession is a curious and imperfect process. Many things take a great deal of effort. Doctors can tend to get set in their ways and use tools and techniques because they are simply the way things have always been done. Alternatively, occasionally innovations quickly become 'great new hopes' that are soon widely adopted with little justification. As I write about a new philosophy of regenerative medicine, I hope to avoid some of these pitfalls.

As an example relevant to regeneration, I perhaps ought to start by discussing developments in stem cell research. Often still described as the key to reducing the impact of ageing, Mesenchymal Stem Cells (MSCs) are derived from both human and mammalian bone marrow and periosteum tissues found in joints. They were first isolated in the 1990s by the late eminent scientist Dr Arnold I Caplan. Caplan is described as the godfather of stem cells as he, together with colleagues at Case Western Reserve University in Cleveland Ohio, not only discovered stem cells, but immediately recognised their therapeutic potential.

Caplan published an acclaimed paper[6] that told the world MSCs appeared to maintain their ability to form new tissue when expanded in cultures outside the body. 'Mesenchymal' became too much of a mouthful and the term 'stem cells' was coined. The prevailing wisdom, at least in orthopaedics, became that stem cells could help reverse degeneration by being grown into bone and cartilage.

Stem cells: What's in the name?

Stem cells, it seemed, were building blocks that could be steered, as they developed, into cells to replace a patient's lost tissue like-for-like. This was obviously very exciting to anyone interested in regeneration and anti-ageing. Millions of dollars were spent on research, momentum grew and soon multiple institutes and thousands of scientists were looking at stem cells to treat any number of conditions and complaints.

Some twenty years later, Caplan, however, back-tracked from his initial assertions and admitted a flaw in his original thinking in a second paper.[7] MSCs had been mischaracterised during his initial research. Caplan urged the medical world to change the name of MSCs to 'Medicinal Signalling Cells'. In the body, they do not regrow as differentiated new cells. They do not change. They cannot be steered. Rather than replace damaged cells like-for-like, they simply act as messengers to prompt other cells to grow. Introducing stem cells into a joint, for example, may prompt existing cartilage to grow thanks to chemical signalling, but it won't create anything new. This effect is clearly less impressive and useful than Caplan's original hypothesis promised.

It seems that medicine's inability to give up on particular dogmas means that the stem cell story continues, undaunted by the changing science. In my experience, many medical professionals in orthopaedics still rely on Caplan's first paper to justify research. Few, it has to be said, seem to have read his second corrective paper and changed track accordingly.

Caplan's stem cell research also introduced another dogmatic idea that is still common in modern orthopaedics – the use of microfractures. The thinking behind microfractures is that drilling a tiny hole in a bone lets marrow, rich in the right kind of cells, escape to aid healing. Again, born in the 1990s, the orthopaedic community came to believe that when a bone starts bleeding, the 'stem cells' within the leaking blood reform as cartilage. This technique was developed alongside arthroscope-enabled keyhole joint surgery. We were, for the first time, starting to see cartilage damage up close and personal without the patient undergoing major surgery. We saw it heal around bleeding bones and a new treatment was born.

There is, however, no real evidence that microfractures make any long-lasting positive difference at all. We know that bone heals because new bone cells form a soft callus that hardens and knits broken sections together. It makes no sense that this process has any impact on cartilage and yet we've been drilling microfracture holes for years. It is an approved treatment on many private medical cover policies and is sanctioned by the UK National Institute of Clinical Excellence (NICE). It has become something surgeons 'just know' and, like all dogmas, everyone just keeps doing as they have always done.

While I am discussing dogmatic thinking that should be challenged, I ought to tackle the prescribing of steroids for joint pain. Steroids are so alkaline that they can be as toxic to humans as acid. If you go to see a doctor with joint pain, however, they are very likely to suggest a cortisone injection to relieve your symptoms without much thought. Actually, nowadays, doctors don't necessarily do the injections themselves. A physiotherapist or another primary carer may end up wielding the syringe. Whoever does the injection, steroids kill a lot of cells as they go about reducing inflammation and pain. A moment's consideration of the long-term balance of regeneration and degeneration in our bodies and you can see this is problematic. Indeed, many reviews and scientific papers have proved that cortisone (a steroid) shouldn't be used to treat arthritis. This is covered in more detail later in the book, but suffice it to say I find it troubling that we continue prescribing steroid injections and ignore evidence that contradicts perceived wisdom and countless medical textbooks and training sessions.

I am not saying, incidentally, there is never a reason to drill into bone or have a steroid injection. A small hole might be useful to create a foundation of new bone as part of a wider joint repair, for example. Careful use of steroids might form part of a considered pain management plan. All I am doing here is suggesting that applying basic scientific knowledge and logic rather than dogma to medical decisions might be a good idea and highlighting the fact that this might mean challenging the status quo.

I will finish this chapter with a tale of two doctors from history that demonstrates this point perfectly. Joseph Lister, a nineteenth-century surgeon from Edinburgh, is widely credited with being the first doctor to link handwashing with patient care. He realised women in his care were dying during childbirth because surgeons went from patient to patient and often between the hospital's operating theatre and morgue, spreading infection as they went. His 1867 article in the *British Medical Journal*, titled 'On the Antiseptic Principle in the Practice of Surgery' literally changed the world.[8] Scrubbing up has been standard practice for surgeons ever since.

This is not, incidentally, a piece of science that needs particular medical knowledge or experience. Lister looked at the evidence and deduced cause and effect. It is actually a classical piece of systems engineering – a subject we will look at in the next chapter.

Lister, however, was not the first person to conclude that dirty surgeon's hands were costing lives. Austrian doctor Dr Ignaz Philipp Semmelweis had spotted the same pattern in maternal mortality at least twenty years before Lister. Specifically, he noted cases of puerperal fever, a form of septicaemia, could be cut drastically if doctors washed their hands in a chlorine solution before gynaecological examinations.[9] Semmelweis' observations, however, clashed with the established scientific and medical opinions of the time. Rejected as an eccentric failure, he died in 1866 in a public insane asylum aged just forty-seven. He never knew he would eventually be proved right by Joseph Lister.

I share this tale to reinforce the importance of proof and sound scientific thinking as you age. You have to be sure before making any changes in your life that they are right for you. This may seem surprising advice considering my profession, but trusting doctors will only get you so far. I would urge you to apply robust science, engineering and design principles to your own ageing process. This will mean you can be confident in any treatments you choose. As a result, they are more likely to work.

This applies from the very start of any process you go through whether it's surgery, chemical treatment or biological therapy. Beginning with an ill-thought-through, unproven 'wonky' foundation will mean everything that follows will be 'wonky' too. Floor upon floor. Storey upon storey. You will be in danger of your plans collapsing all around you.

Summary

I urge you to step back and ask yourself: 'Is my thinking straight? Do I trust the advice I'm getting?' Remember, the medical consensus is not always correct. We, as a profession, often defy logic and simply follow dogma because it is what we've always done. We ignore things we disagree with and don't necessarily read papers that correct scientific errors. In the mid-nineteenth-century, we thought Dr Ignaz Philipp Semmelweis was insane when he asked doctors to wash their hands. What do we know?

I am hoping that, despite the multiple challenges solving the complex problems ageing well presents, you are feeling inspired to take the next step, which is to approach the problem systematically.

THREE

Mechanistic Versus Systematic Thinking

N ow that I have discussed the taxing nature of problem-solving in today's regenerative medicine, we ought to move on and consider what shifting our thinking might mean in practice. How does it help us become superhuman? How does it help us regenerate?

For example, many of the orthopaedic surgeons I know are sometimes guilty of treating joint pain as a simple problem with a simple solution. In doing so, they are often over-keen and enthusiastic to view replacement surgery as the appropriate treatment. They tend to focus on their technique. Improvements are often framed by making surgery faster and more efficient rather than, perhaps, more effective for the patient. I understand this view. I am an orthopaedic surgeon myself, of course, but I have learned the value of occasionally challenging the assumption that surgery is always the best treatment. There are, as we will see, more regenerative options to consider. What counts, when you're looking for the best answer, is how you frame the question.

Imagine you live in a simple country dwelling and need some firewood. If you take an axe and hit a tree trunk with sufficient force, you will get your firewood. The problem is simple. There's one input (the tree) and one output (the firewood). The process of chopping the wood is mechanical. Now, imagine you are faced with a patient with knee pain that you want to alleviate. By viewing this as a problem with just one input (a painful degenerated joint) and a single output (the implantation of a pain-free metal and plastic replacement knee that replaces degenerated natural tissue), you are describing a mechanical process. You are engaging in mechanistic thinking.

When problems become complicated, you may be forced to introduce a series of interim steps between input and output. Turning your tree into flat-pack furniture provides a good example of this because, as we discussed in the preceding chapter, flat-pack furniture is typically supplied with an instruction manual. Helpfully published by the manufacturer, such instruction manuals describe the solution in an easy-to-follow sequence: step one, step two, step three and so on. Taking this illustration further, installing the components of a modern sports car engine, for example, is far from simple as a task. Still, it would be theoretically possible for anyone to do it with detailed instructions to follow. It need not, actually, be a human process. Modern car production lines have been based around sophisticated robots for many years now. This is because machines are ideally placed to slavishly follow the same pathways time after time. Machines will always get the same results. Some view orthopaedic surgery in the same way and the automation of more of our tasks cannot be far away. The problem with this future vision is it still depends on mechanistic, rather than systematic, thinking. It assumes the problem is a simple one.

Complex problems, in comparison, have multiple inputs, multiple outputs and multiple interdependencies in between, which means each situation is unique. It is worth parking analogies and illustrations here to give you a commonplace example directly from my experience of regenerative medicine. Creating platelet-rich plasma, for example, from patients' blood is an unpredictable process. You can spin a centrifuge to concentrate red blood cells thousands of times without ever getting the same result. Treating a patient using a concentration of platelets that is too low won't have the desired effect. Too high, and there is evidence you might end up doing more harm than good. It is akin to Goldilocks tackling the bears' porridge. Is it too hot, too cold or just right? As the input varies every time the process is completed, a simple instruction manual or robot would be of limited use.

This is why, when we look at regenerative medicine in particular, we should not solely rely on tried and tested mechanistic approaches. We need to think about solving the many regenerative problems systematically.

Zooming out

We can, and do, look at the body in various ways – both as doctors and patients. You might tell me your elbow hurts, for example. I will, of course, investigate. I might feel, scan or X-ray your elbow joint, but what exactly am I looking at? The dictionary tells us the 'elbow' is simply the joint between the upper and lower arm. Indeed, you could view it as a simple hinge point between bones and if you're experiencing elbow joint pain, it is perhaps reasonable to assume that is where the problem lies. A doctor, based on your description, might start down familiar orthopaedic routes for treatment.

If we are thinking regeneratively, however, there is limited use in viewing any joint in isolation. It is more useful to view an elbow joint as a more complex system than a simple hinge in, and of, itself. For example, your elbow comprises three bones: the ulna, the radius and the humerus. A total of twenty-three muscles are directly associated with the elbow joint's movements, including flexor, extensor, flexor-pronator and extensor-supinator groups. There are the ulnar, median and radial nerves and their branches to consider too, as well as your bicep and tricep ligaments and tendons. It is, of course, also part of the body's wider musculoskeletal system, which, in turn, is part of the whole body's immeasurable complexity. Based on this simple description of the elbow alone, it is perhaps easy to see the value of 'zooming out' and taking a broader, holistic view of musculoskeletal problems before making any treatment decisions.

You would think, given the rapid development of medical technology, that taking a broad holistic whole-body view is becoming less challenging. I'm not convinced this is the case because, alongside today's innovation, there seems to be a growing trend for specialisation. Medical professionals are becoming experts in ever smaller and more discrete aspects of our trade. The generalist is increasingly being replaced by specialists and subspecialists. This undoubtedly brings benefits to an individual's chosen fields of study but, on the downside, can lead to reductionist thinking overall. Any system can be broken down into components. Each component can be studied in ever-increasing detail. This might, however, not always be in a patient's best interests. What if the whole performs differently than the sum of its parts? Where does the overview lie? Who, among the myriad of experts, has the whole picture?

In a fascinating paper, 'Osteoarthritis: A Disease of the Joint as An Organ'[10] published in 2012, Dr Richard Loeser and others argue that describing osteoarthritis, the most common form of joint pain, as natural wear and tear affecting our bones is unhelpful. The paper compellingly argues that osteoarthritis is better, and more usefully, described as a disease character-ised by abnormal remodelling of joint tissues driven by inflammation. The degeneration of bone is, in fact, only one of the factors that may cause it. This leaves plenty of other causes that may be treatable with non-surgical therapies. The paper's conclusions ought to encourage doctors to resist the mechanistic temptation to rush to surgery.

To return to our painful elbow, it follows there are a couple of things to consider before deciding on a partic-ular course of treatment. Firstly, it is important to have a clear idea of how the joint is performing as a whole system. Secondly, it is important to understand its posi-tion within the body's wider systems. This shouldn't feel radical. To successfully treat the musculoskeletal system, we simply need to look at joints in the same way medicine looks at the rest of the body's organs. Taking cardiology as an example, it is a foolhardy sur-geon who rushes to a heart transplant before taking a view of the whole of a patient's cardiovascular system.

Zooming out to a system-wide view will, I trust, lead to more imaginative treatments being offered to patients. Given the increasing range of options available today, it seems a shame so many of today's patients are simply asked to choose between pain relief and joint replacement surgery. Yes, the results of the latter can be impressive, but is it always in the patient's best interests overall? We are more likely to be able to answer that question correctly if we 'zoom out' and take a wide, systematic view of the problem.

Establishing a baseline

All regenerative medicine needs a purpose. Orthopaedic professionals typically spend their days with people who want to be in less pain and improve their mobility. The goals will vary from patient to patient, but we are used to managing patient expectations and setting realistic treatment goals. Most of the time, we know where we are going and we can imagine a future for our patients. However, we don't always have clarity around where we are starting from.

Take elite footballers as an example. If you'll forgive a sweeping generalisation (look away, Peter Crouch fans), the best footballers often have bow legs – a condition known medically as genu varum – which sees the legs naturally curve outwards. The more bowed a footballer's legs are, the shorter the player tends to be and the closer their centre of gravity is to the ground. This makes them more difficult to tackle as they run and dribble the ball. A curved leg is also better for generating horizontal forces when passing or shooting. Horizontal forces are better for speed and accuracy than vertical forces.

Strikers who can hit the ball along the ground with force are more likely to beat a goalkeeper and less likely to hit the crossbar. We can see bow legs, on average, make turning and twisting past opponents and scoring easier and, it follows, we have demonstrated that they are probably an advantage to a footballer. Yet we also know bow legs overload the inside of the knee joint and stretch the outside, which can cause instability, pain and, ultimately, arthritis.

Bow legs present sports science with a medical dilemma. For a successful player, at the height of their powers and earning potential, fixing their bow legs to prevent painful knee joint degeneration might cost them the skills that make them successful. How best to treat a professional footballer, then? For many, unfortunately, the answer is simply to wait until they retire before they take their knee problems seriously. By this time, the pain is often worse and the treatment required is more dramatic. For those who can't wait, we have to think beyond the obvious and perhaps start treatment from a different angle.

Although bow-legged footballers illustrate the problem neatly, every patient needs to negotiate an individual balance between the impact of treatment and the likely outcomes. What outcome would they consider a success? What are they willing to do to get there? 99% of the discussions I have with my patients are about 'getting back to normal'. The inherent difficulty of discussing musculoskeletal health is that the definition of 'normal' is different for everyone.

The problem isn't quite the same in other branches of medicine. For major surgery, it is standard practice to measure haemoglobin levels in a patient's blood as part of the pre-op routine. The results provide a 'normal' benchmark doctors can use after the operation to see how much blood a patient has lost and if any action is required to get back to healthy levels. Compared to complex musculoskeletal treatments, this is ridiculously straightforward. We can, however, borrow the principle of creating and referring back to a 'snapshot' of a healthy body. Using this concept, we can perhaps define the task of any regenerative treatment plan as returning the patient's mobility to an agreed prior baseline of healthiness.

If our football player was a star in the penalty area able to bury the ball in the back of the net, then regenerating his knee should, arguably, take him back there. In elite sports, analysis, data, modelling and even TV footage can be brought together to create a picture of an athlete operating at their best relatively easily.

However, unfortunately for the rest of us, we do not routinely record, or even pay particular attention to, the healthy performance of our musculoskeletal system. We are not conscious of how our muscles and joints feel when they are working well. It all happens subconsciously. We take it for granted and simply crack on with our lives. We certainly do not, as a rule, X-ray ourselves when we are healthy. MRI scans are so expensive that they are generally only available as a diagnostic tool to people investigating serious symptoms.

There is one discipline we can use to get a baseline, though. We can all observe how we move using Newtonian mechanics. We can see how we respond to force and acceleration. The observation needs no specialist skills at all. It may, in the past, have required specialist equipment, but today most of us carry devices that can take a baseline snapshot of how we move pretty much every time we leave the house. A short film or movie, simply recorded on your smartphone, provides a snapshot that might prove incredibly useful if you find yourself in muscular pain. It provides a baseline you, and more importantly, your doctors, can refer to in the event of compromised mobility. It needn't be complicated, but a niggle that might be hard to describe or replicate during a consultation can be obvious on film. A film of you standing from a sitting position gives us a huge amount of information.

I often ask both professional and amateur runners to film themselves in action on the road or track. Runners tend to push the body to its musculoskeletal limits all the time and so small changes can have big implications. Where movement might normally be smooth, a film might reveal something jolting or out of line that it would be easy to miss otherwise. This is probably a good moment to mention that motion has a ripple effect, sometimes known as the kinetic chain. A problem with a runner's hip, for example, might affect their knee, which, in turn, may cause the spine to twist and damage the shoulder, for example. Studying motion on screen makes it easier to see where the ripple begins. It also, as an aside, shows why zooming in and narrowly focusing on a single issue when patients present pain can often be costly.

It is also worth reiterating that everyone has a unique baseline of healthy movement. Every musculoskeletal system is a complex mix of levers, hinges and joints and, genetically identical twins aside, no two assemblies are ever precisely the same. Christened a 'kinematic signature' by some, the way you move is seen to be as individual as your fingerprint.

The sophistication of this kinematic science is growing incredibly quickly. Cutting-edge orthopaedic and musculoskeletal medicine already has access to marker-less motion capture technology that can accurately track natural movements. AI diagnostic software can help analyse the results too. There may be a future where we all have a perfect, detailed digital record of our healthy movements filed away somewhere in the cloud ready for when it is needed. Until then, shooting and saving a video clip of you standing from a sitting position on your smartphone is probably a sensible move. *If the goal of regenerative medicine is a return to normal mobility, what could be more helpful than a record of what normal looked like for you in the past?*

Thinking like an engineer

To demonstrate what I mean by thinking like an engineer, I'm going to suggest, again, moving away from medicine briefly. If, over the summer, you have ever put a temporary paddling pool out in your garden for your kids to splash about in, you will know you inevitably have to sacrifice a patch of grass underneath it. When the summer ends and autumn comes, you will be faced with an unsightly patch of bare dead lawn. How do you respond?

You may be a keen gardener. You might begin to research which grass seeds to buy, start planning the feeding and watering regime and wonder how you'll explain to the kids that they can't play on that bit of ground until next spring. How about keeping your pets away from the area too? It's a big old task. There's no time to waste. An engineer, in comparison, will probably begin by calmly checking that the paddling pool has definitely been removed and packed away. You can have the greenest fingers in the world, but if you miss the first critical step of a job, your best-laid plans will have no impact whatsoever.

This is a fun example often told by engineers to amuse themselves and catch out the unwary. I am slightly biased, having spent six years studying medical engineering leading to a PhD in the subject, but I like it too. It is a great illustration of the way engineers think and I am convinced it is the kind of thinking that will help improve the outcomes of regenerative medicine.

As I studied at my School of Engineering, I became more and more immersed in engineering's grounded, pragmatic and practical problem-solving culture. I was impressed by the fact that, compared to medicine, their approach to finding answers came more from logic, learning, rules and principles rather than from textbooks and case histories. I ought to say I have no wish to discard or dismiss medical practice or even necessarily criticise it. The knowledge we have all gained from our medical training and traditions is vital, as is continual medical research, innovation and collaboration. I am simply suggesting there are gains to be had, particularly in regenerative medicine, from combining a medical view of the world with engineering's step-by-step approach to undertaking tasks.

To see what a combined medical and engineering approach might deliver in practice, let us look at a common musculoskeletal example. Common orthopaedic practice tells us painful knees can often be fixed with an operation known as meniscectomy. Meniscectomies typically involve a surgeon trimming away damaged meniscus tissue. Healthy meniscus tissue forms crescent-shaped pads that provide a cushion where the human femur and tibia bones meet.

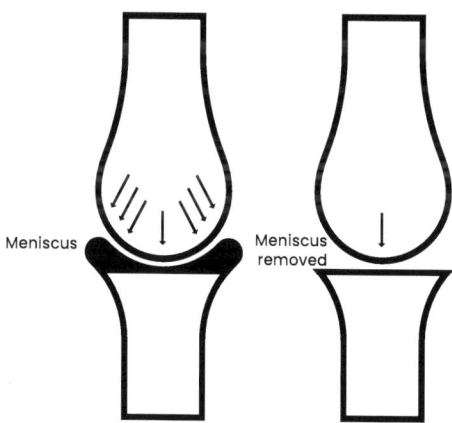

The meniscus and the ball of the femur and the flat of the tibia

The menisci act as vital shock absorbers between the round ball of bone at the top of our femurs and the flat surface of our tibias. Without menisci, the femur's ball simply skids and grinds against its flat tibia counterpart. You can no doubt see why this leads to pain. As well as the grinding and skidding, there is point loading to consider. When you put weight through a knee joint with healthy menisci, there is an additional surface area to spread the load. Without cushioning, all the pressure goes into a single point, making the joint weaker and more susceptible to damage.

Faced with a bad, torn or ripped meniscus, undertaking a meniscectomy operation to remove, or trim, degraded tissue is often an orthopaedic surgeon's first instinct. It is what the medical textbooks have said to do for years, after all. Surgery might fix the immediate problem but leaves the knee with less cartilage. The way the joint handles loading will be affected too. Both these things can lead to further joint degeneration in the long term. Despite short-term pain relief, with a meniscectomy operation, you can risk increasing the chances of arthritis in later life.

What is an engineering approach, then, to a painful knee? Where does it differ from a traditional medical response? If we remember that, before buying grass seed in the autumn, a good engineer will check if the paddling pool the kids played in all summer has been removed, it is important to understand the knee problem from first principles without making assumptions. Engineers zoom out and take a whole systematic view of the knee and its wider role.

It may be that removing some, or all, of a patient's meniscus cartilage is still necessary. Engineers, however, understand a simple mechanistic approach might just lead to more problems down the road. The additional knock-on procedures may reflect changes in the Newtonian physics of the body. A knee might need to be realigned to better manage the forces running through it. This might mean additional surgery in the form of an osteotomy procedure to change bone alignment. A similar effect might also be achieved using external bracing. We might look at ways to repair menisci rather than removing them. We could encourage cartilage cells to regrow or start anew. We could look to chemistry and biology with drug or hormonal therapies. More physics-based treatments might involve employing electromagnetism to energise cartilage cells to prompt their regeneration. The list is long and, thanks to the rapid development of new technologies, is getting longer all the time.

Summary

Today, when it comes to fixing a painful knee, or any other musculoskeletal issue for that matter, we have more options in our toolbox than ever before. This is fortunate because, as we've established in this chapter, musculoskeletal degeneration is a complex problem and finding answers for patients means adopting a methodical, systematic approach. This means, sadly for the medical profession perhaps, doctors and surgeons cannot act like robots. We cannot repeatedly follow the same set of fixed instructions to treat our patients. Like engineers, we have to learn and apply a set of principles to each task and methodologically work through a huge series of options to find the right treatment.

Now, if I've succeeded, you are looking at ageing from a different perspective. If you're excited about thinking systematically like an engineer, it is probably time to move away from theory into practice and start designing. In the next chapter, I start on the first of my four pillars of the regeneration principle: physics.

Action points

- **Apply Science and Engineering**: Utilise scientific methods and engineering principles to approach regenerative health challenges.

- **Time Interventions Wisely**: Recognise the importance of timing in therapeutic interventions for optimal regeneration.

- **Incorporate Sports Science Insights**: Leverage advancements and innovations from elite sports science for broader medical applications.

- **Question Medical Conventions**: Be open to challenging established medical dogmas to discover more effective regenerative solutions.

- **Personalise Your Regenerative Path**: Design a bespoke regenerative health journey based on individual needs, informed by scientific evidence.

FOUR
Physics

The three preceding chapters set out my regenerative arguments and principles. I think now it is probably time to start talking about specific applications of regenerative medicine. This is where we start learning how to become superhuman. Where better to start than physics? Not only is it the science behind Superman's flight and the Hulk smashing things up, it is the oldest of our academic disciplines. If you include astronomy as one of its branches, it is arguably as old as human civilisation itself. The first documented astronomical observations, for example, date back to the Assyro-Babylonians over 3,000 years ago.

Put simply, physics is the study of nature's forces and the phenomena that cause them. Perhaps the most obvious example of a force that impacts every aspect of our existence is gravity. It is a constant presence that exists throughout the universe, but despite centuries of study, we have yet to come close to understanding its cause. We do, however, know an increasing amount about its behaviour. Over the summer of 2023, for example, US scientists proved the existence of background low-frequency gravitational waves, potentially caused by neutron stars orbiting black holes, passing through Earth.[11] The insight that gravity behaves like light, among other things, proves Einstein's theoretical discoveries were right on the money.

There are, of course, a myriad of other forces to study and explore, from the nuclear forces that hold atoms together, to the thermodynamic forces that boil water to make our cups of tea. Physics, as a discipline, keeps growing in scale and complexity as humanity continues on its quest to understand how the universe works. Even idle reading on our latest discoveries and theories can, however, quickly become a mind-bending reminder of how little we know and how insignificant we, as human beings, are in the grand universal scheme of things.

This is why, you'll be pleased to know, I am keeping this chapter firmly grounded in medical physics and, specifically, the physics involved in regenerating the musculoskeletal system. I will leave 'multi-universe theory' and 'the God particle' to others and focus on the forces that your bones, muscles and joints experience throughout our lives.

Newtonian physics takes its name from Isaac Newton, who is possibly most famous for first formulating the theory of gravity in the mid-seventeenth century. Legend has it he surmised what forces were at work when an apple fell out of a tree. True or not, it makes a good story.

Understanding the musculoskeletal system and the forces that act on it as we go about our business is perhaps the major factor in regenerative health. It's easy to be healthy if you stay still, motionless and unmoved by the world. In reality, we are all constantly in motion from the moment we get out of bed and bend to pull on our socks every day. It is all explained by physics.

Newtonian mechanics

Newtonian mechanics describes the study of how, and why, things move. In the world of musculoskeletal medicine, it describes how our bodies react to physical forces. Like everything else in the universe, any human activity, from a tennis serve to a ballroom dance, is governed by Newton's three famous Laws of Motion:

1. An object at rest remains at rest, and an object in motion remains in motion at constant speed and in a straight line unless acted on by an unbalanced force.

2. The acceleration of an object depends on the mass of the object and the amount of force applied.

3. Whenever one object exerts a force on another object, the second object exerts an equal and opposite force on the first.[12]

One way to view our bodies is as a collection of masses connected by levers, hinges and pivots that have evolved over millennia to keep us alive. Providing we are safely on earth, gravity continually pulls us downwards with a constant force. For those interested in numbers, this force is 9.81 Newtons, with one Newton being defined as the force required to accelerate one kilogram at the rate of one metre per second, every second. This is the force that acts on us when we're standing still. As we walk, momentum means we push down through our joints with a force between three and eight times greater than normal.

1st Law	2nd Law	3rd Law
F ●→ V Then V forever or at rest forever	F V a F = ma	F1 → ← F2 F1 = F2

Newton's law of motion

We are generally, of course, rarely conscious of gravity acting on us. We only feel gravity's effects when we fall or jump off something. This isn't something we're born with, though. Any parent will remember the tears that come as a baby begins to toddle and comes face to face with this aspect of life. It is the acceleration due to gravity described by Isaac Newton's work that makes landing painful.

Whether we are aware of them or not, Newtonian forces cause wear and tear every day of our lives. To understand degeneration, we tend to look at the way we walk. In modern-day life, we sit a lot too, go up and down stairs and lift and carry things. As an aside, we like to think that going up and down the stairs rather than taking a lift is the healthier choice. In Newtonian terms, however, it isn't necessarily a good thing. We'll discover my views on the 'great lift or stairs debate' later in the book.

All our actions – walking, running, jumping and climbing – put our knee and hip joints under significant pressure and can accelerate degeneration. Once a joint is painful, it needs to be protected from forces running through it to heal. We have all been told not to put weight on a strain or break. This 'unloading' is key to successful musculoskeletal regeneration and repair. One way of achieving this is to brace a joint. In recent years, exoskeleton-style products that can brace a joint are becoming more popular and increasingly sophisticated. Exoskeletons have always been a feature of sci-fi stories and movies. They often give characters superhuman strength and abilities. In the real world, applying a carefully designed form of bracing to the body can certainly change how we respond to forces applied to it. There are many different types of offloading or unloading braces available. They are all, however, a non-invasive treatment that uses the theory of Newtonian mechanics in practice to protect joints. They can have an incredibly positive impact on the speed of recovery from damage and disease. Removing damaging forces is the equivalent of removing the paddling pool discussion from the preceding chapter and an elegant example of thinking like an engineer in action.

Once a force is removed, healing might happen naturally. In many cases, all that is required is time. In other cases, we still need to provide some form of treatment. This could be muscular strengthening through physiotherapy and exercise, which is still very Newtonian in nature. Repeated action against a force such as stretching or lifting has an impact on our muscular strength and can restore a joint's functionality. If exercise doesn't help, there are other treatments that we'll consider in later sections. They're straying away from Newtonian physics, but in a perfect regenerative world, these should all be considered before surgery.

Once surgery is required, it, too, relies on Newtonian physics. As an example, let us consider a high

tibial osteotomy operation. It fixes knee misalignment which can develop through disease or injury.
Misalignment causes further tearing and degeneration of the joint's menisci and articular cartilage. As
a result, knee bones grind, bump and knock painfully
when put under force. A surgeon undertaking a high
tibial osteotomy uses the principles of Newtonian
movement to unload the damaged area of the knee
joint by cutting and wedging the upper joint. The procedure can realign the bone to ensure that forces act
elsewhere. Before committing to a knee replacement,
we can also implant devices into knees that act as
shock absorbers. Again, this is using Newtonian principles to manage how forces apply within the body.

It is not just knees, of course. The whole skeletal
system needs protection. Of all the areas that can be
affected as we age, perhaps the most important is
our backs. An elite tennis player, for example, might
put forces equivalent to twenty times their body
weight through the facet joints that link the bones
of the spine. This overloading causes two problems.
Firstly, the joint will become inflamed. The beauty
of muscle, however, is that with rest and treatment,
inflammation can be reversed. The body will recover.
The joint will regenerate. It can become stronger
than it was, and you can then afford to put it under a
little bit more pressure. An amateur tennis player's
back might strengthen through practice. However,
if you keep on abusing your body as a professional
on the tennis circuit, there will be no time for this
recovery. You can go past the point of regeneration

into degeneration and cause damage that the natural healing process can't help with. This is why athletes turn to medical science. Chemical and biological treatments are important and can always help the body recover, but it is mechanics that drives everything. When it comes to sports medicine, physics is number one.

Let us return to the knee, specifically the knee cap, to illustrate why. We were given knee caps, or patellas, so that we can stand, walk, run and squat efficiently. They are the flattened oval bones that sit on the front of our knee and act as a lever arm. They exist so that when your muscles pull on the longer bones in your lower leg, your tibias, your femurs (or thigh bones) act as levers and you lift your hips.

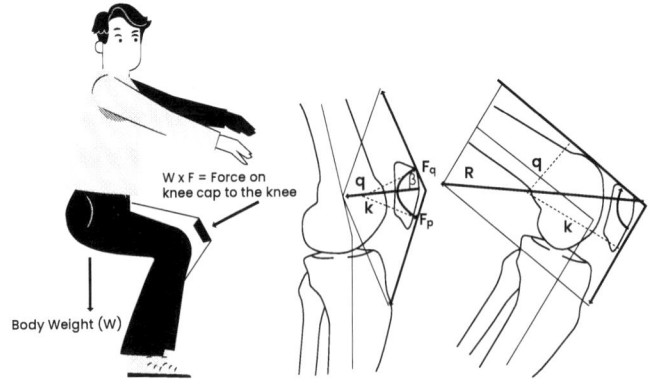

Knee cap biomechanics

Your patellas, it's fair to say, have a tough time of it with a lot of forces to contend with. The table below illustrates how our activities can put a force up to twenty times our body weight through them. Considering how small patellas are, they truly are superheroes.

Forces on the patella for a 70kg person

Motion	Force in Newtons[13]	Percentage of body weight
Walking	350 N	½ body weight
Biking	350 N	½ body weight
Up stairs	2,450 N	3.5 times body weight
Down stairs	3,500 N	5 times body weight
Running	5,000 N	7 times body weight
Squatting	5,000 N	7 times body weight
Deep squatting	15,000 N	20 times body weight

There are countless other examples of mechanics at work in our bodies. Much of it goes unnoticed because it happens without us having to think about it. We would struggle to stay balanced without the extra corrective leverage our big toes give us at ground level, for example. Our collarbone doesn't appear to do very much but, sitting at the top of our spine, it allows our shoulders to handle large rotational forces. If you hold something with your hand with a straight arm and no midpoint to rest on, you'll soon feel the pressure there.

It is clear our anatomy has been designed, or at least evolved, to be efficient. We are generally good at walking on two feet, running, holding and throwing things. You can see our prehistoric roots in our system and find clues to our earlier history as a species too. I sometimes find myself referring to my veterinary colleagues and pondering how we used to move on four legs. We may have more in common with our furry ancestors than, perhaps, we like to admit.

Overall, we spend a lot of time talking about Newtonian physics. As a discipline, it is over 350 years old, of course, so it feels familiar and established. It is something most of us learn at school and Newton's three main laws of motion ought to at least ring a bell. It is the second law that has the biggest impact on our musculoskeletal health:

Force = mass × acceleration (or F = ma)

In general, we try to minimise forces running through our body. Less force equals less pressure and less pressure equals less pain. Even standing still, we are under gravitational force. As we move, acceleration adds to the force. Increased mass, or weight, adds to forces too. This is why we often ask our patients to lose weight.

Lifting and carrying things is another way to add mass to the equation. By carrying a load and putting extra rotational forces through the shoulder, for example, people can suffer from muscle pain in the neck, the trunk and even the hand. This is physics in action.

The maths is compelling. Only 10% of extra force going into a joint, whatever the reason, for five years potentially adds up to 10,000 times the force that should be going through it. It is easy to see why degeneration can become a problem.

Despite the fact that physics appears to be a wholly scientific affair, when it comes to musculoskeletal health, our observations can often still be subjective. For example, three medical professionals could watch a patient walk on a treadmill and identify three different problems. The good news is thanks to modern scanning technology and diagnostic software, we are getting closer to more accurate objective diagnoses all the time.

You can also help yourself, of course. We discussed recording a baseline earlier in the book. Having a record of your body's healthy responses to the forces that act on it might prove useful should things go wrong. You might look a bit odd filming yourself walking, running, sitting and standing, but it'll be worth it.

My final tip related to Newtonian physics is to replace your shoes regularly, especially if you're a runner. Even a few centimetres of worn-out sole can have a significant Newtonian effect on how your feet, knees and hips operate.

Electrical muscle stimulation

If you've ever had an electric shock, even a minor one, you'll know electricity can have quite an effect on your body. You probably know that our hearts beat because of the electrical signals applied to them too. It is the reason we use an electro-cardiogram test to check everything is in working order. If it's not, we sometimes use defibrillators to shock the heart back into action.

Electricity, however, has an impact on all of our systems. It is how our body communicates. Fine, small electrical currents, measured in milliamps, travel between our nerves sending messages and prompting action. It is electric pulses that cause our muscles to contract and release. If you see a cartoon character stick its fingers in a socket, you'll no doubt see an amusingly exaggerated version. Introducing electricity to the body from the outside is normally bad, dangerous and best avoided. However, when it comes to the musculoskeletal system and regeneration, we can use it to our advantage. We can carefully use electricity to help us contract muscles we cannot move ourselves. This is either because they are damaged, or sometimes prolonged damage means we have forgotten how to. The main use of electrical forces in musculoskeletal regeneration is the stimulation of muscles. A little shock can help the body remember neuromuscular connections, rebuild nerve fibres and start the process of returning muscles to normal action.

To do this we use a device known as an Electro Muscle Stimulation device, often shortened to EMS. An EMS uses a slightly higher shock than similar pain-reducing systems to actually cause muscles to twitch – shortcutting the brain and nervous system. We can get a weak muscle to contract and release repeatedly without asking the patient to do anything consciously. If, for example, a lateral thigh muscle has been weakened by injury, electrical therapy can kickstart the healing process and strengthen it before we ask the patient to do lots of exercise and physiotherapy.

The other way we use EMS technology is postoperatively. Following surgery muscles, cartilage and tendons can need waking up. They've been cut into and damaged, after all. Electrically induced movement doesn't hurt the patient, but the muscles are still active. Electrical treatment will reestablish healthy neurological pathways and start recovery more quickly than the patient can manage alone.

Electro muscle stimulation devices are unsurprisingly common in professional sports. Some athletes use them as a specific training pathway. They can be targeted to specific muscle groups, so cyclists may employ it on their thighs before the Tour de France, for example.

For most of us, however, EMS is something you'll use to regenerate a muscle group that may have become weak through illness or injury. One area that using an EMS certainly won't help with, however, is losing weight. I'm sorry to report it pays to be incredibly cynical about the EMS devices that market themselves as tightening up 'tums' or giving you a six-pack. In reality, you already have a six-pack. If you can't see yours, it is due to the fat hiding it. Stimulating muscles won't shift that.

A few milliamps of electricity applied in the right place can, however, certainly help with muscular regeneration. You can buy devices to help you at home relatively inexpensively too. It's certainly worth a try.

Electromagnetism: scanning and therapy

Electromagnetism is another of nature's fundamental forces. Electromagnetic waves form around electric currents and, while interactions with the body are not widely understood, it is useful in a handful of medical applications. The most common is arguably the MRI scan. MRI, standing for Magnetic Resonance Imaging, refers to a non-invasive method of producing internal images of the body. It works by using electromagnetic and radio waves to align molecules in the body. The molecules in different parts of your body, such as bone and cartilage, for example, will align differently. The MRI scanner can spot these differences and turn them into diagnostic images. Excitingly, the latest developments in MRI scans use AI and machine learning to automate their interpretation. By studying more MRI results than a doctor could ever dream of, AI can learn to spot diagnostic correlations more accurately than a mere human could ever achieve.

Other applications of electromagnetic fields are not as well researched but have been shown to have therapeutic effects. There are plenty of theories from simple copper bracelets to hugely expensive 'proton treatments'. With all of them, I'd advise caution. That's not to say there hasn't been excellent research into regeneration over recent years. Electromagnetic waves have been shown to potentially enhance healing in both animal studies and a handful of human clinical cases. Applying different electromagnetic waveforms and patterns can, it seems, prompt positive changes in cartilage, muscle and bone.

The beauty of treatment by an electromagnetic field is that it's an external procedure. You don't feel a thing. We established earlier that even with electricity, you feel your muscles twitch, which can feel uncomfortable. With electromagnetism, it just works. It doesn't, however, work immediately. Electromagnetism needs a slow, low release to be safe – let alone effective. The energy needs to go into your body as a pulse. This is why an MRI scan can take forty-five minutes compared to less than a second for an X-ray.

Given that it is at the cutting edge of treatment, I would not necessarily advise using any electromagnetic treatment products at home. Without professional medical advice, it is easy to fall for empty marketing claims rather than enjoy sound, well-researched evidence-based treatments. From what we know already though, the future of electromagnetism for muscle, bone and joint regeneration looks incredibly exciting.

Ultrasound treatment

Ultrasound has woven itself into the fabric of modern medicine. You may recognise it from the delicate task of guiding new life into the world through neonatal scans or the precise shattering of gallstones without surgical intervention. In the domain of musculo-skeletal health, its role has been largely diagnostic. It offers a window into the complex world of tissues and bones through sending and recording the echoes of sound waves. It is a silent observer, revealing tears in tendons and the delicate patterns of cartilage as it heals and weaves back together.

Yet, today the scope of ultrasound stretches beyond diagnosis. Therapeutically, it's evolving at an ever-increasing rate. A gentle hum can be used to massage muscles buried deep within our bodies. The psoas muscle, for example, is nestled in our pelvis against our core structural elements and surgically inaccessible. Here, ultrasound can regenerate muscle. It is generally gentler than the more overt call of electrical therapies discussed earlier.

Extracorporeal Shock Wave Therapy (ESWT), a particular type of ultrasound therapy, has emerged as a notable recent innovation. As the name suggests, it uses targeted sound waves, or 'shock waves' to carry energy to painful musculoskeletal tissues, rather like the ripples from a stone thrown into a pond. These waves convert to heat and mechanical energy upon contact to cause microtraumas that stimulate blood flow and prompt cellular repair. This is effectively using sound to coax tissues into a state of healing. It's a fascinating interplay of physics, biology and energy transformation combined therapeutically. Unlike its brutal cousin, the defibrillator, which jolts life into a faltering heart with electricity, ESWT nudges the body's tissues gently towards repair with sound.

Wave-based therapies are generally growing in importance as they are non-invasive and focus on enhancing the body's innate healing response. Waves, through their energy, initiate a cascade of biological responses that lead to the regeneration of bone and soft tissues. They essentially 'massage' our cells, encouraging them to rebuild and renew.

Low-level laser therapy

In the world of regenerative medicine, light has recently provided big steps forward in the form of laser beams. What could be more superhuman? At the right frequency, laser light can cut through tissue with amazing precision. It is much more accurate than our usual surgical tools, but lasers do more than just cut. They can also pass through the walls of our cells unnoticed at certain frequencies.

A blast of the right laser light can give cells a regenerative boost without causing any harm. This can help cool down inflammation and get the body's own regeneration going. This means that, when it comes to arthritis and long-lasting pain in muscles and bones, laser treatments are being increasingly seen as a helpful treatment option. They work on a very small scale, changing how cells act by using very specific types of light. Low-Level Laser Therapy (LLLT) is especially good for easing stiffness and pain, thus accelerating healing.

A lot of research has been done on LLLT's impact within damaged knees. This has shown the benefits go beyond pain relief to helping the body start to heal from the inside. We are still figuring out all the ways LLLT can help, but it's clear that it has a lot of potential. It's a time when old health problems are being met with new, high-tech treatments. As with any new medical treatment, it's important to stay updated with the latest research and to listen to medical advice. The field is always changing as new things are discovered. For doctors and patients, knowing the most recent information is crucial, so that the steps we take for better health are based on solid science and careful medical advice.

It's crucial to remember that physics is more than just forces acting on our bodies. It encompasses a range of elements like electricity, light, sound and magnetism, all interacting in complex ways with our physiology. Light therapy, especially in the form of lasers, is a prime example of how these physical elements can be harnessed for healing and regeneration. This chapter underscores the idea that our understanding of physics can profoundly impact medical advancements, offering new and innovative ways to approach health and healing. By exploring the intricate ways in which various physical phenomena like light interact with our bodies, we gain a deeper appreciation of their potential in regenerative medicine, reminding us that the principles of physics are not just abstract concepts, but vital tools that can aid in our journey towards better health.

Summary

As this chapter dedicated to the role of physics in regeneration draws to a close, it's essential we acknowledge the broad spectrum of physics. While Newtonian physics remains a cornerstone in regenerative medicine, particularly in surgery that corrects mechanical issues, it is always just one piece of a larger puzzle.

Other branches of physics, encompassing electricity, light, sound and electromagnetism, are perhaps subtler in their impact and require more time to manifest results, yet they are equally vital. These therapies give us precision incisions by laser, healing prompted by the rhythm of sound waves and more. They act as additional tools in our armoury and enhance our regenerative potential. Each patient presents a unique scenario, necessitating a tailored approach where these diverse elements can be balanced and applied judiciously.

By delving into the interactions between various physical phenomena and our bodies, we unlock new possibilities in health and healing. These explorations in physics do not exist in isolation. They are integral to the ongoing journey of enhancing regenerative medicine, reinforcing the notion that physics, in all its forms, is not merely theoretical but a practical ally in our quest for optimal health and wellbeing. Physics is one of our superpowers.

FIVE
Chemistry

The word chemistry often conjures up evocative images of white lab coats, mysterious liquids, changing colours, acrid smells, Bunsen burners, bangs and indecipherable equations scribbled on chalkboards. This is certainly how the subject is typically represented in Hollywood. Many a superhero's origin story involves a chemistry experiment going wrong. While these images are still very much part of the subject, the scope of modern chemistry as a discipline reaches far beyond laboratory walls. It is intricately woven into the fabric of our lives and, more specifically, how our bodies degenerate and regenerate. Chemistry keeps us balanced as we grow, age, get injured and repair ourselves. We can certainly say that at any given time, the adage, 'You are what you eat,' could be extended to, 'You are what you're made of,' chemically speaking.

In this chapter, we will move on from physics and delve into the world of organic and inorganic molecules, compounds, chemical processes and treatments that apply in today's regenerative medicine. Modern medicine is increasingly leveraging chemical principles to better repair damage and amplify our interventions. Thanks to our increased understanding, we are better placed than ever to use chemistry to protect our musculoskeletal system from damage and pain and accelerate regeneration and healing.

So how does chemistry help us, exactly? In the case of organic chemistry, it forms the very building blocks that make up our bodies. It is carbon-based molecules that form *all* the compounds we need to live, including carbohydrates, proteins, lipids, nucleic acids (DNA and RNA) and more. If you were to think of your body as a sprawling metropolis, then organic chemical structures would be the bricks and mortar, the electricity, the transport system, the sewage system and even the citizens going about their day. It is organic chemistry that creates the environment in which all our physiological work gets done.

Elements that are not carbon-based, or inorganic, such as sodium, potassium, calcium, fluoride and iodine also have a vital role to play in shaping the body's chemical environment. Take calcium for example. Not only is it a structural element in our bones, it plays a vital additional role in our musculoskeletal system by serving as a signalling molecule for a range of cellular functions, including muscle contraction.

Both inorganic and organic molecules are involved in the delicate balance that keeps us healthy. We have used the body's chemistry medically for many, many years now. While we might not have understood the functionality at the time, ancient plant-based remedies from our ancestors have their roots in chemistry. For a more modern concrete example, consider the local anaesthetic. Typical local anaesthesia works by injecting specific chemical compounds that block sodium channels to our neurons. These, in turn, prevent the propagation of any nerve impulses. Any pain signals are chemically, rather than physically, cut off at the source.

How do we manage our body's chemistry in everyday life? Some of the ways are obvious. We might suggest a course of drugs. We might also recommend a change in diet, including taking any number of supplements. Hormone treatments also affect the body's chemistry. Even more prosaic lifestyle changes such as reducing stress levels, getting more sleep and spending time outdoors in the sun can have a measurable chemical impact.

In regenerative medicine, chemistry is an area that has, perhaps, historically been overlooked in the rush to fix problems using other disciplines. This is especially true if you compare it to the Newtonian physics favoured by orthopaedic surgery and discussed in the previous chapter. However, more of us than ever have an understanding of the potential of chemistry-based regenerative treatments. Today, it represents an exciting new source of innovation. In the rest of this chapter, I'll share some examples of chemistry at work right now.

Cartilage cell regeneration

I developed my thinking around chemistry while working in the laboratory during my Medical Engineering PhD. I was fortunate enough to have a lot of time to explore cells and the environments they operate in thanks to access to university research facilities. Of course, the behaviour of cells grown in a laboratory is incredibly straightforward compared to cells growing in the human body. Laboratory cells typically have one role – to multiply so we can study them.

Cell lineage is measured by a passage number which records the number of times the group of cells, or culture, has been harvested and reseeded into multiple sub or daughter cultures. Passage 0 refers to the origin, the first generation that grows exponentially through the natural process of mitosis (ie, division into two identical nuclei). This culture can be split to form a new set or culture of cells known as Passage 1. This can be repeated ad infinitum leading to Passages 2, 3, 4 and so on. In this way, the original becomes father, grandfather, great-grandfather and so on to countless daughter cells. Rates vary between cell types, but I've seen some human cells double in volume every hour under laboratory conditions. This exponential growth and ability to reproduce is ideal for growing replacement tissue to help us regenerate damaged joints.

A great example of this in practice is the Autologous Chondrocyte Implantation (ACI) operation. This is a surgical procedure that has developed a track record of good results over the last twenty years using new cells to treat damaged cartilage in the knee. It can ease pain, swelling and restricted movement. The first part of an ACI procedure involves harvesting healthy cells from a non-weight-bearing area of the knee joint surface. We can then break these cells down to their purest form: chondrocyte cells – the only source of cartilage we know of. These are cartilage's 'Passage 0', the granddaddy, the start of all the cartilage structures in our joints. Once harvested from the patient, the building blocks can be replicated exponentially outside of the body in the laboratory. The patient, typically three to five weeks later, undergoes a second procedure using an arthrotomy or an 'open joint' procedure to implant the newly grown daughter cells and, potentially, repair any degraded or damaged cartilage.

A problem with chondrocyte cell implantation as a technique today is that we implant cells into the body straight from the laboratory. We ask cells that have been grown outside the patient to affect an established highly complex system in the body. A knee joint, for example, is a unique environment to each and every patient. Without tailored cells, implantation can feel a bit like shooting in the dark and merely hoping to hit the target.

We are not there yet, but we'll soon be in a position to shape cells by chemically altering a cell's growth medium in the petri dish. By changing how cells grow and giving them the correct signals, we can deliver personalised outputs from the same source. This will allow us to create more targeted help, including growing bone and muscle tissue. If I was malevolent (which, fortunately, I am not), I could even make cells cancerous. Whatever the goal, the outputs of cell growth are increasingly under our control.

This, however, comes with a big caveat. At present, any understanding we have of biochemistry has mainly been gained from experimentation and a lot of trial and error. Our assumptions are based on laboratory work where we can control a lot of things, rather than within the body where our influence is more limited. The future, however, looks exciting.

Platelet-rich plasma

In the realm of regenerative medicine, the use of Platelet-Rich Plasma (PRP) therapy is an example of harnessing the essential elements of organic chemistry to repair our bodies. The process begins with a simple extraction of about 10 millilitres of blood from the patient. Once outside the body, this blood undergoes centrifugation to separate its components and isolate blood platelets enriched with growth factors like PGF (platelet-derived growth factor) and cytokine proteins. These factors are not just cellular components; they are the very messengers of healing, directing cells towards repair and regeneration. Injecting this

PRP back into an injured area is like sending a bio-chemical SOS, signalling the body to commence its natural regenerative processes.

The complexity of PRP therapy is fascinating. PRP isn't just a single entity, but a spectrum of formulations, each with its unique characteristics and potential. This diversity covers levels of white blood cells (leu-kocytes), protein-rich and protein-poor variants and activated and non-activated forms. Even the speed of centrifugation makes a difference to the platelets' properties.

Despite this, PRP therapy remains a relatively straight-forward example of regenerative chemistry in action. We extract, we separate, we concentrate and we rein-troduce. It provides a concentrated dose of healing potential right where it is needed. The magic lies in the centrifuge. This acts almost like an alchemist's tool, spinning out the less useful elements and leav-ing us with potent healing compounds.

This makes the centrifuge itself central to the pro-cess. It's more than a machine; it's the core of PRP preparation where the interplay of gravitational and centrifugal forces, timed precisely, is crucial in shap-ing the efficacy of PRP. Mastering the centrifuge's operation is akin to conducting an orchestra. Each minute adjustment is vital to achieving the perfect blend of platelets and growth factors and pivotal in transforming PRP from a simple blood derivative to a finely-tuned therapeutic agent. It is no exaggeration to say PRP preparation embodies a point where scientific precision and artistry meet.

PRP's versatility is further enhanced when it is mixed with other chemicals or substances to augment its inherent properties. For instance, combining PRP with hyaluronic acid (which we'll cover later in this chapter) can provide a more robust framework for tissue regeneration. This ability to blend and adapt compounds makes PRP therapy an intricate science. It demands great technical expertise, but also a deep understanding of the biochemical processes at play.

The application of PRP is not without its debates and variations. The concentration of platelets, the method of activation and the injection technique – all these variables play a role in the efficacy of the treatment. The science behind PRP has evolved, leading to different formulations like Standard PRP, A-PRP (Activated), B-PRP (Biotin-enhanced), and C-PRP (Combination PRP), each designed for specific regenerative needs. These are not just variations, but strategic adaptations to harness chemistry for healing.

We can see that PRP therapy, in its various forms and combinations, represents more than simple medical treatment; it is a testament to the regenerative power and potential of organic chemistry. Yet, PRP is not a panacea. It works best in concert with the body's overall health and mechanical functionality. It is part of a broader strategy, not a standalone miracle cure. As we delve deeper into regenerative medicine, we understand that PRP is a single chapter in the larger story of superhuman healing.

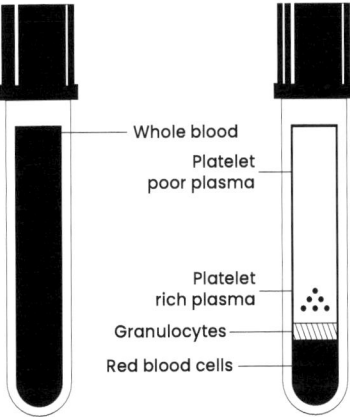

Platelet-rich plasma

Platelet-rich fibrin

Further into the regenerative medicine chemistry book, we encounter Platelet-Rich Fibrin (PRF). This is a biomaterial that takes the principles of PRP to the next level. PRF is still derived from the patient's own blood but, as the name suggests, adds fibrin to the mix. Fibrin is an insoluble protein formed as blood clots. It creates a scaffold-like structure that aids in the migration and proliferation of cells and, as a result, acts as a veritable cradle for healing. The role of PRF in cartilage repair and regeneration is underscored by its unique composition. It's not just a healing agent, it's a biological architect. It shapes the way cells repair and regenerate damaged tissue.

Clinical evidence points to PRF enhancing the quality of cartilage repair, particularly when used in conjunction with stem cells.

Alongside cartilage regeneration, its use is being explored in other medical fields. Given its ability to create a personalised healing environment, PRF is leading the way to truly tailored regeneration processes that match each individual's unique biological makeup. Through this, we are exploring a new chapter in the story of regenerative medicine. We'll soon be in a world where a patient's own biological materials are used to maximise healing and minimise risks. It's a step towards a superhuman future where treatments are not just applied, but crafted to fit us all perfectly.

Exosome treatment

Platelet-rich plasma and PRF work on a macro level in the body. Despite their exciting potential, such treatments still depend on pumping blood into a joint to kick-start healing. It's relatively unsophisticated and there are many, many more nuanced tools we can use from the body's chemistry to help us regenerate at a more nano level.

Exosomes, known as extracellular vesicles, help us by acting as signalling molecules, for example. They are the mechanism by which cells communicate with each other from the granddaddy at Passage 0 to the descendants of, say, Passage 10. Information and instructions are shared between cell generations through exosomes in the same way family wisdom might pass from parent to child. If the PRP injection treatment described above provides a simple headline signal to start healing, *exosome treatment is more akin to providing a textbook on how to heal.* Exosomes use our body's messenger ribonucleic acid (mRNA) molecules to pass on advanced knowledge.

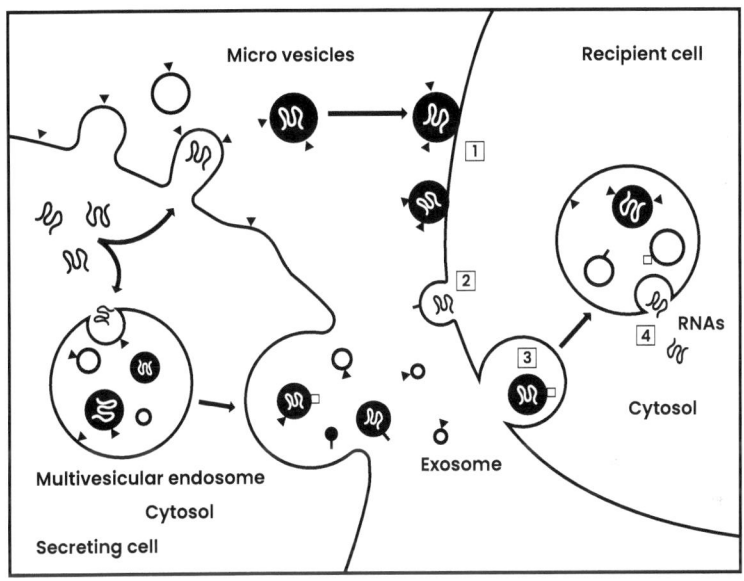

Exosome

With exosome treatment, we can do more than instruct cells to start regeneration. We can tell cells how we want them to proceed. This makes exosomes an exciting new frontier of regenerative medicine. At present, however, there's no way of producing the amount of unique exosomes that we need from one patient. This is why, today, we pool donated exosomes from a range of sources. This isn't as effective as it could be. Further work is still in an experimental phase, however, and it won't be that long before we're generating exosomes more selectively and creating specific chemical guidance to cells that matches an individual patient's needs.

Hyaluronan injections

The treatments we have discussed so far in this chapter have been examples of organic chemistry in action. However, regenerative medicine also has a place for inorganic, man-made solutions. They come into play mainly when we move away from fixing an issue to maintenance. For example, we can use our knowledge of how cartilage is built to help protect it over time. There are two relevant basic building blocks within cartilage itself: a form of carbohydrate known as glycosaminoglycans (GAG) and hyaluronan, also known as hyaluronate or hyaluronic acid. The third option, incidentally, is rarely heard in treatment rooms as the word 'acid' rarely sounds good for us.

Hyaluronan is a compound within our extracellular matrix (ECM) that regulates tissue responses during injury, repair and regeneration. The good news is we can make it in the lab. You might have heard of hyaluronan because dermatologists and skincare brands have a range of uses for it based mainly on the fact it is great at retaining water, thus protecting the skin by preventing it from drying out.

Of course, the collagen in our joints has the same need to retain water because dry cartilage degenerates quickly and painfully. The key thing about hyaluronan is that it can be man-made to suit specific purposes in the body. A smaller hyaluronan molecule might be used as a filler to iron out wrinkles in the face. A larger molecule can be injected into a knee, for example, to ease lubrication in the joint. Think of it as a form of WD-40 that will keep the joint free of friction and allow it to move a little better.

Hyaluronan doesn't just act on the joint surface. It also has a positive impact on the connective tissue, known as the synovial membrane, that lines the inside of the whole joint capsule. In a healthy joint, synovial fluid fills a bubble around the joint to keep everything lubricated and flexible. Hyaluronan stimulates the production of this liquid.

Injecting hyaluronan works as an effective treatment by changing the chemical environment within the joint as a whole. Typically, when we use it, we are changing the environment within the synovial membrane to give cartilage cells more water. This, in turn, lubricates movement, prevents wear and tear and minimises pain. This makes hyaluronan a great inorganic chemical treatment to have in our armoury to maintain musculoskeletal health.

Polyacrylamide gel (PAAG)

Polyacrylamide gel, known as PAAG, is another man-made chemical treatment that can help joint regeneration. In some ways it fulfils a similar role to hyaluronan, however, it is more complex. It acts like silicon gel rather than a simple lubricating oil. It lasts longer and has more of an anti-inflammatory effect than other treatments.

PAAG is a combination of water and carefully designed synthetic linear polymers that mimics the natural synovial fluid within a joint. It also, thanks to its molecular structure, has a unique fire blanket effect on inflammation. This is because it has large molecules that act as inorganic chemical barriers that actively block communication between inflammatory cells.

When a joint is inflamed by arthritis, for example, it feels hot and angry. PAAG has an ongoing calming and dampening effect that suppresses the ability of pain to spread. This means it is an alternative to painkillers, anti-inflammatory drugs and corticosteroid injections, which only offer temporary relief. PAAG provides a physical barrier on the lining of the joint and also cushioning and support in the joint, directly addressing the mechanical aspects of degeneration.

This can work alongside physiotherapy and exercise to strengthen muscles around the joint, improve mobility and reduce pain. Polyacrylamide gel treatment has, in this way, proven to considerably delay the need for joint replacement surgery by a good number of years.

PAAG is a non-biodegradable permanent implant that won't necessarily improve a joint's health, but will prevent symptoms from getting worse. You can see it as a chemical intervention that slows down degeneration. It's a man-made, inorganic injection that alleviates the symptoms of chronic musculoskeletal damage and is increasingly common as a treatment for arthritis, particularly among former elite sportspeople. Former sports stars often struggle with joint decay at a relatively early age when they are, otherwise, in good overall health.

In the case of one patient, a former Olympic swimmer in her fifties, PAAG proved decisive when stiffness and pain in her right knee was identified as Grade 4 arthritis. She chose non-invasive, single injection PAAG treatment because it offered long-lasting pain relief, delayed the need for surgery and allowed her to lead the fully active life she had grown used to. This, according to the patient, had as much of a positive impact on her mental wellbeing as it did physically. As sport and fitness had been such an important part of her life, being able to keep active was especially valuable. This is a useful reminder that although we are often talking about micro- and nano-level interventions when we are describing chemical treatments, we are always treating the whole patient.

Steroid injections

Another inorganic treatment for the symptoms of musculoskeletal issues is the steroid injection. Typically cortisone, steroid injections have become a very common treatment for joint pain. Unlike the inorganic chemical treatments above, however, there is a growing body of evidence that this choice is actively bad for you. It is demonstrable that steroids ultimately damage cartilage. Despite relieving pain, they kill cartilage cells, harm your joints and contribute to musculoskeletal degeneration.

I can say this with a degree of confidence based on the work of the Cochrane Library, an international not-for-profit network that publishes independent peer reviews across the health sector. As an example, their paper 'Corticosteroid Injections For Shoulder Pain'[14] finds multiple references to poor data, small and short-lived effects and little overall benefit when it comes to steroid injections. A quick browse through similar reports shows this is representative of steroid musculoskeletal treatments as a whole. Patients report feeling free from pain because the steroid compounds do reduce inflammation. They do this by influencing multiple neurological signal transduction pathways. Put simply, they switch off the effects of inflammatory genes, but they do not affect the root causes.

Doctors continue to give steroid injections because of their short-term benefits and ignore the long-term consequences. A major problem is that steroids are typically over a hundred times more alkaline than normal pH levels in the human body. This is enough to destroy structures within a joint, including nerve cells. Steroids, however, are ingrained in orthopaedic dogma and training as granting immediate pain relief. Sports people often rely on steroid-based treatments to get back on the pitch pain-free and at an accelerated rate. This may work but comes at a cost – the pain is masked but any damage remains.

Steroids, therefore, should only be used in very specific circumstances. For example, a low dose can reduce pain and inflammation, giving the patient some respite, while the root cause of a problem is investigated. Given its destructive qualities, however, it should never feel routine or be done simply out of habit. You sometimes hear of a treatment plan involving six-monthly steroid injections from a physiotherapist or GP. In my mind, this is not regenerative medicine; it is actually the beginning of the end. If anything, it's hastening degeneration and too high a price to pay for any short-term relief.

Summary

In wrapping up our exploration of chemistry's role in regenerative medicine, it's vital to revisit the overarching principles of physics, chemistry, biology and timing that underpin regeneration by design. Chemistry stands as a crucial pillar in this framework, offering direct means to influence the delicate balance between regeneration and degeneration. The interplay of organic and inorganic chemistry in medical applications exemplifies how we can enhance regeneration, temper degeneration and return the body to homeostatic stability.

A useful illustration of this idea in action comes in the form of treating osteitis pubis in elite athletes. This is painful inflammation in the groin area caused by inflammation in the joint between the pubic bones. It is an area that is largely inaccessible to surgery and neatly illustrates the limits of physical intervention. When surgical options are limited, multidisciplinary approaches involving alternative treatments typically become welcome.

It is here that the benefits of treatments such as PRP and hyaluronan injections are easy to see. These, and other chemical interventions, can help alter the environment within the affected area, stabilising it and aiding rehabilitation. They can then alleviate pain and restore movement. The success rate of chemical treatments for osteitis pubis speaks volumes about the potency of chemical interventions.

I trust we've proved that chemistry, though it may not always be as prominent as the mechanical aspects discussed in physics, is far from a secondary player in the realm of regeneration. As highlighted in this chapter, innovations like PAAG implants showcase the burgeoning potential of chemical treatments. These implants, responsive to the body's condition, offer joint stabilisation and present a viable alternative to more invasive surgical procedures. This, and the other tools we've touched upon, are evolving rapidly. This promises a future rich with groundbreaking advancements. As we delve deeper into biochemistry, our strategies are likely to become more effective, more nuanced and more aligned with our body's natural processes. The road ahead in chemical regenerative medicine is one of discovery and innovation.

SIX

Biology

Having covered physics and chemistry in the preceding chapters, it probably won't come as a surprise that the next superhuman regenerative building block is biology. In particular, we will look at the specific biological processes and treatments that affect the human musculoskeletal system and its regeneration. There is, inevitably, a significant cross-over with chemistry. Indeed, the subject is probably more accurately described with the one catch-all term: biochemistry. However, I think there is value in separating the two disciplines and giving biology discrete attention it might otherwise miss out on.

In discussing biology, it is definitely worth reiterating the point that everyone is different. Every single member of the human race has a body that is wholly individual and highly complex. This is largely due to genetics, of course. Everyone starts life with their own, singular never-to-be-repeated DNA road map. It is, however, also true that every single one of us leads a different life and will experience different external influences. Work, play, diet, exercise, psychology and countless other issues all have a hugely significant impact on our bodies. A middle-aged hard-drinking deep-sea diver, to choose an extreme, if unlikely, example, will have a very different biology to a young vegan beach volleyball player. The choices they have made and experiences they have had throughout their lives will have shaped every aspect of their biology. With this in mind, whenever we think about biology and regenerative medicine, we need to think of our patients' lives, history, wants, needs, expectations and limits. Where have our patients been? How have they lived? What environments have they operated in? What circumstances suit them the best? The answers, biologically speaking, will be evident in every aspect of their physiology down to cellular level: the building blocks that make up our bodies. What environment have cells developed in? What do cells need? What will make them flourish? What will regenerate them?

Such questioning is closely linked to the big philo-sophical question about the meaning of life itself. Despite our best efforts, modern technology and rap-idly increasing scientific understanding of biological principles, we still do not completely understand how to define life. Indeed, we cannot agree on what 'living' actually means. To be morbid, briefly, if we study a person moments before and moments after death, their biology, chemistry and physics remain pretty much unchanged. We routinely study human embryos, but can't put our finger on the moment they stop being a group of cells and become living people. When exactly does the spark we have come to call life begin and end? Science has yet to find a precise answer.

Pondering the nature of existence and consciousness, however, reminds us to think about life systematically when considering regenerative medicine. We always need to think of the subject as part of the wider picture that makes up a patient's whole being. We need to view their biology as an incredibly complex set of interconnected processes. Even if we do not understand it completely, we ought to always consider health and well-being overall and in the round.

To help, let us imagine an elite tennis player's serve again. Perhaps it is at match-point at Wimbledon, the culmination of the player's whole career. In an incredibly high-pressure moment, every single component of the player's body is likely to be in action and focused on delivering the ball to the other end of the court as quickly and accurately as possible. Any discrete treatments the player has had mean little now. His medical team might have treated his elbow mechanically, by strapping it perhaps. He might have had electro-muscle stimulation on his thigh a month ago and chondrocyte cell implantation in his knee the year before, but they are just parts of the picture. Many, many more factors, including the player's biological processes, will influence whether the critical serve is a success or failure.

Although we tend to pick on key dramatic moments in our lives, the same concept of interconnectedness is key to our health overall and day-to-day well-being. Biological processes and treatments play a vital role for every one of us in ways we are not even aware of.

Circulation, electricity and kinematics

There are several examples of biological interconnectedness directly relevant to regeneration. The first, and perhaps most obvious, is the circulatory system that distributes blood to every corner of our body. On the face of it, the primary function of this system is the delivery of nutrients, oxygen and energy. Our hearts beat to pump vital ingredients around the body from calories we have ingested to oxygen we have inhaled.

Our blood, however, does more than carry raw materials. It also plays a key role in communicating between our cells, organs and systems. Cells within it carry signals from one part of our body to the other. This is why we routinely have blood tests as part of any checkup we might have from our doctors. We have learned to interpret some of these messages and, by careful analysis, we can use them to spot early signs of disease and deficiencies in nutrients and minerals. Biological messages can also tell us if our liver is functioning normally, our kidneys are working correctly and so on. The circulatory system is an information superhighway.

As discussed in the physics chapter of this book, we also know our bodies communicate through electrical signals. We can measure them too through routine tests. Electromyograms (EMGs) show us how a patient's muscles twitch in response to neurological stimulation. This can tell us a great deal about the performance of muscle tissue. Electrocardiograms (ECGs) are, perhaps, more familiar and show doctors how the heart is responding to the brain's electrical prompts to continue, one hopes, beating correctly.

Again, we learned through physics that our bodies communicate a great deal through how they move. In regenerative medicine, the complex processes of motion are often referred to as the kinematic chain. We can use the study of motion, or kinematics, to spot changes in the performance of joints and limbs. For example, we can identify knee and hip problems by simply watching how a patient moves from sitting to standing. Elite sports performers routinely analyse how they run, take a shot, throw a javelin, bowl a cricket ball or any other technique to gain an insight into how their body is dealing with the movement, forces and impact involved.

Through understanding biological principles and how the body operates, doctors and sports scientists can identify potential problems or opportunities for improvement and competitive advantage. The science of kinematics is rapidly developing thanks to Musculoskeletal Action Imaging (MAI) technology. This innovation combines state-of-the-art imaging with AI diagnostic tools to build highly detailed and accurate pictures of human biology in action. This may soon replace using the human eye and subjective interpretation from doctors or radiologists with objective, quantifiable machine learning. Imagine a future where an Artificial Intelligence, that has learned from millions and millions of cases, analyses how your musculoskeletal system moves, provides quantifiable feedback and objectively suggests treatment.

Collagen injections

Collagen is the main biological building material in our bodies, which is why I have chosen to discuss it in the biology chapter rather than the earlier chemistry chapter. It forms the bonding material, known as connective tissue, that keeps us together. It is the material that connects cells and creates the environment that we ask our cells to operate within. If our body's connectivity and our cells' environment are not in optimal condition, it does not matter what treatment we propose, nothing will regenerate well. We need the right building blocks in place. We need healthy collagen for anything to improve.

To date, science has discovered fifteen types of collagen in human biology. I'm confident we will find more as our understanding of cells and cell behaviour increases. Of the fifteen, we mainly use two in musculoskeletal medicine. They are conveniently known as Type One and Type Two. Type One is primarily associated with our bones. Type Two is pretty much anything else including our skin, muscles, organs and tissues. The other thirteen types of collagen fulfil various specialist roles in the body, but make up a tiny proportion of the total in our systems.

The elasticity of the collagen changes as we age. This is why our skins get a little bit flabbier, our bones get more brittle and the 'shock absorbers' in our joints get harder and less flexible. This is why movement gets challenging as we age and we become prone to damage over time. We discussed the behaviour of cells as we age in the first chapter of this book, but cells degenerate over time and become slightly less efficient in processing collagen. All this means the quality of collagen, the vital connective tissue of our body, can leave a lot to be desired as we age and our systems degenerate.

The good news is the quality and amount of collagen can be altered in the body through various interventions. It can be taken as a supplement. There is strong evidence, for example, that ingesting collagen supplements has a positive impact on the elasticity reported in patients' skin. It is, less scientifically, possible to see the results by looking in the mirror at our faces.

The same measure, elasticity, is harder to prove on the inside of the body, but similar positive results are reported. The best kind of collagen supplement is derived from fish. Fish collagen is absorbed significantly more efficiently into the human body than alternatives. It is worth noting that plant-based alternatives are also widely available on the market today.

We can also supplement the body's collagen by injection. Here, I am referring to local treatment rather than generally intravenous delivery of collagen through the circulatory system. This may happen in the future, but today, we have the technology and know-how to directly inject and implant collagen into specific areas of the body: a knee joint, the pelvis or between vertebrae, for example. These direct interventions have a proven track record when it comes to improving the environment in which we ask cells to regenerate within. As a result, they are an increasingly common biological tool for professionals involved in musculoskeletal repairs.

Vitamins

Vitamins are important ingredients that are useful to enhance the building blocks of the human body. Vitamins are organic compounds that operate in a similar way to enzymes. They enable and accelerate a range of processes in the body, including the production of collagen. Without vitamin C, for example, it doesn't matter how many collagen supplements you take, they are going to be processed inefficiently.

There is evidence for this in history. Scurvy, the infamous disease reported among Elizabethan sailors during long voyages, was eventually diagnosed as a vitamin C deficiency. There was almost no understanding of nutrition at the time, of course. Sailors with no vitamin C in their diet for years at a time became unable to process collagen. Without this ability, they experienced a range of disturbing systems, including chronic fatigue, excruciating joint pain, muscle wastage, sores, spots, skin blemishes, bleeding gums and missing teeth.

Nowadays, mercifully, we understand the value of nutrition and most of us get sufficient vitamin C to avoid scurvy through mixed, healthy diets. It is common, however, for doctors to suggest vitamin C supplements for patients who need a collagen boost. Alongside vitamin C, vitamin D is very useful for bone health as it helps the body process calcium. In fact, one of the causes of osteoporosis as we age is a lack of vitamin D in our diets. We also create vitamin D from direct sunlight on the skin when outdoors. An afternoon of sunbathing can help our bones, who would have thought? If a patient requires supplemental calcium, it is normal to suggest additional vitamin D at the same time. The body simply won't absorb the first well enough without the second.

Vitamin E is an antioxidant that is extremely good for the skin. It helps it retain its elasticity while eradicating some of the free radical molecules that can cause damage to skin cells. Vitamin A is very good for our eyesight. This is thought to be where the old wives' tale about eating carrots helping you see at night comes from. Vitamin B helps the neurovascular system and our hair. In fact, vitamin B is often successfully included alongside PRP in regenerative treatments for baldness.

Vitamins can work wonders for our biology. Healthy levels can normally be ingested through balanced diets that include the right mix of fruit and vegetables. Those needing a bit more help might take them as supplements. In some cases, they can be intravenously injected too. The latter is generally considered more efficient as it bypasses the gut. Many elite sports people regularly take vitamins through intravenous injections or a drip to maximise their impact. This, however, also needs some care. Mishandled, intravenous vitamins may get absorbed by the kidneys and passed straight out of the body through our bladders – wasting a lot of effort.

Hormones, exercise and sleep

Hormones are also an extremely important part of the regenerative package. We have all heard of examples – testosterone, progesterone, melatonin, endorphins, growth hormones and cortisol are all in the mix. The exact composition varies by gender, age and ethnicity, but also our life choices and experiences. We all end up with a unique, delicate hormonal balance that changes over time.

With this in mind, most of the time we experience hormones as effective, good and helpful parts of our biological makeup. There are circumstances, however, when they get out of balance, go awry and have a negative impact. They tend to operate in a cyclical way that is linked to a wide range of factors, including our levels of happiness, how we cope with stress, our reproductive systems, our sleep patterns and even how much natural light we get. Hormones, and how they behave, play a vital role in how we regenerate. The impact of hormones varies, but they cause changes in our systems from the microcellular level through to the operation of our major organs such as our heart and lungs through to our brains.

Looking specifically at musculoskeletal regeneration, hormones such as Human Growth Hormone (HGH), for example, are responsible for triggering the creation of new proteins that replace damaged ones in muscles, tendons and ligaments. As an aside, these hormone levels are typically highest during sleep, so enjoying a good night of shut-eye is often an important part of regeneration.

Testosterone in men and its relationship with exercise might also prove a useful illustration of hormones at work. Testosterone levels peak after men have exercised. After a good workout, men will experience a surge of the masculine sex hormone that is responsible for the generation of typically male physical characteristics such as muscle mass, strength and the growth of facial and body hair. As part of any recovery process, testosterone influences parts of the cell cycle that support regeneration. Not all exercise is the same, though.

Cardiovascular fitness is generally defined by repetitive, dynamic movements that raise heart rate and enhance lung function. The most common type by far is distance running, but the list also includes cycling, swimming, aerobics, rowing, stair climbing, hiking and most types of dancing.

The pinnacle of cardiovascular workouts is surely running a marathon. Its notable elite runners of both genders are generally very lean. Indeed, in races, they tend to burn their fat and carbohydrate reserves in an effort to win. They are depleting their bodies rather than regenerating them. What is more, running can exacerbate pain and damage to joints due to repetitive impact forces. It really is the wrong type of exercise to grow muscle. It also has a significantly smaller and more short-lived impact on testosterone levels than the alternative – strength, resistance and weight training associated with weightlifting, for example.

Exercises that centre on static or controlled movements against resistance will definitely help regenerate our muscles and joints more effectively than going for a run. In men, they are also associated with higher levels of testosterone, which adds to the regenerative effect. This is possibly why the stereotype of hyper-masculine weightlifters increasingly growing muscle mass feels so familiar. Food, training and natural testosterone add up to their familiar physiques.

It is worth noting that women do have smaller amounts of natural testosterone in their bodies that may have a similar effect on muscle mass. Progesterone and oestrogen have different effects on joints and muscle mass. There is some evidence that progesterone and oestrogen, for example, help women regulate muscle mass and strength. Progesterone also promotes bone growth. It is also notable that osteoarthritis is often associated with the drop in female sex hormones that occurs during menopause.

The other hormones associated with exercise are endorphins. Often linked with the 'buzz' of winning, endorphins are released whenever we are feeling happy and have been directly linked to pain relief. We instinctively know that stress, anxiety and depression are bad for us and yet we naturally seem to focus on negativity in our lives. It is important not to forget the positive impact that joy, happiness and pleasure can have on our health.

The endorphins released when we are feeling good have a direct impact on our regenerative health.

They act as a trigger to release nitric oxide into our blood vessels, for example. This compound relaxes and opens up blood vessels, improves our circulation and makes us more receptive to growth. It is the ideal state for regeneration. Nitric oxide also reduces levels of our body's natural stress hormone, cortisol. We are probably all familiar with the damage stress can cause, yet we tend to focus on dramatic life events. We all fear heart attacks and mental health crises. In reality, stress builds over time. One big peak of stress can break people down, but when we discuss stress in terms of regenerative medicine, we are generally talking about repeated small doses that slowly and steadily eat away at our biology.

The answer, however, is not to remove stress and cortisol from our systems entirely. We need to feel stress from time to time as it keeps us safe. Cortisol triggers adrenaline and glucose as part of our fight-or-flight response when we perceive danger. It is also the hormone that tells us to wake up in the morning. It keeps our heart beating and helps us control our blood pressure. There is nothing inherently wrong with cortisol. The problems come when it operates when we do not need it to. Timing, as they say, is everything.

Let us take the morning as an example. As it has just triggered us to wake up, we tend to have an excess of cortisol levels during breakfast. This makes early mornings a great time for exercise. Why not use the buildup of our fight-or-flight hormone for something productive? Too much cortisol at night will impact badly on your ability to drift off to sleep. This is why stress is often reported as a cause of insomnia in sufferers. Although it might feel odd, exercising just before bed is a great way to 'work off' excess cortisol and get to sleep.

Rather than trying to remove stress, the best approach, as we have proved, is to try and manage it in sync with our natural rhythms and cycles. Science proves that it also helps to be happy. The release of endorphins that comes with feeling good has a markedly positive regenerative effect. I recommend that all my patients, whatever treatment pathway they may be on, start every day by looking in the mirror and smiling. It is a small and simple, but surprisingly effective tool that works thanks to the complexities of human biology.

Smiling to regenerate

In the fascinating journey of regenerative medicine, one of the most surprising but heartwarming discoveries has to be the power of a simple smile. Smiling, as an instinctive human expression, plays a more significant role in our biology than we might initially perceive. Both spontaneous and deliberate smiling can, it has been proved by multiple researchers, trigger a cascade of neurotransmitters, including endorphins, serotonin and dopamine. These chemicals are not mere mood elevators; they are instrumental in stress reduction and, consequently, in enhancing overall health and the body's regenerative capacity.

We have discussed endorphins in the context of exercise, but even those released during smiling act as natural painkillers. Natural serotonin, another side-effect of smiling, uplifts mood without the adverse effects commonly associated with pharmacological interventions. Dopamine also fosters a positive feedback loop in the brain, promoting healthy behaviours and potentially boosting the efficacy of regenerative treatments. Smiling releases a milieu of biochemistry that indirectly supports regenerative processes by establishing a more conducive physiological environment for healing and tissue regeneration.

Research from the University of Kansas, USA, indicates that smiling during brief periods of stress can lower the body's responses independent of the individual's actual emotional state.[15] This finding is particularly relevant in clinical settings where managing patient stress is crucial for successful treatment outcomes.

Beyond the psychological benefits, the act of smiling has been shown to have tangible biological implications. For instance, research by Kraft and Pressman (2012)[16] linked smiling to lower heart rates during recovery suggesting its potential role in stress mitigation. Fitriana, Santoso, and Dharmana (2020)[17] noted that smiling leads to improved stress responses and the release of endorphins, fostering a positive outlook crucial for recovery and regeneration.

But can smiling actually regenerate tissue? Yes, seems to be the answer when it comes to our eyes. In the context of corneal regeneration, the impact of smiling is noteworthy. Studies, such as those by Han et al (2019)[18] and Zarif et al (2021),[19] have associated smiling with early regeneration of the connective tissue that makes up much of the cornea.

It is worth remembering these findings as you go about your day. The evidence points to smiling being a superpower. Who would have guessed?

DNA and mRNA

As with all living things, human biology is largely defined by our DNA. However, regenerative medicine is not yet at a point where we routinely work directly with a patient's DNA with gene therapies. We are not currently in the business of creating genetically modified material as part of treating the musculoskeletal system. Theoretical and experimental work is certainly moving in that direction, though. One day, I'm sure, DNA treatments will use modified cells to produce highly effective, unique regenerative treatments for every patient. It will, however, take time and some clever science to get us there.

Regenerative treatments are more likely to use mRNA than DNA in the short term. Messenger Ribonucleic Acid is a single-strand helix molecular structure that, like DNA, exists in all of us. It is much simpler than DNA's twin helix because, rather than contain the big, long script that is our bodies' genome, mRNA only contains short bursts of information. It acts as a kind of encryption software that uses specific proteins to communicate at a molecular level. If DNA is an old-school tape, the kind you might have backed up your data with during the early days of computing, mRNA is a much more dynamic and up-to-date technology. It is a WhatsApp-style communication tool that whizzes snippets around the body quickly and efficiently. What makes mRNA useful is we know how to amend it in a similar way to vaccines. We can use it to send any message we want directly into cells' receptors. As well as musculoskeletal therapies, this technique is currently being investigated as a method of treatment for cancers, auto-immune conditions and metabolic and respiratory diseases.

The speed at which mRNA operates, however, comes at a price. It's not very stable. Short and thin, its compounds can soon break down and can only be used at very low temperatures.

With a myriad of practical steps to overcome, it might be a while before DNA and mRNA treatments become more commonplace in regenerative medicine. It is, however, likely that these exciting nano-biochemical tools will become more commonplace and begin to have a major impact soon.

Stem cell treatment

We have discussed the rights and wrongs of the term 'stem cell technology' in the second chapter of *Regeneration By Design*. Although misleadingly mis-labelled, they are still very much with us today. The fact that the term is still in common usage despite the science being disproved provides an example of how dogma can overtake facts and illustrates the dangers associated with treatments becoming fashionable.

Despite being wholly inaccurate, the term 'stem cells' is predominantly still used to describe two forms of cells that are often injected into joints in support of regeneration. The first example is derived from bone marrow. Known as Bone Marrow Aspirate Concentrate (BMAC) treatment, this process sees doctors 'sucking' a patient's bone marrow from a rich source such as the pelvis, spinning it in a centrifuge to create a concentrate and then injecting this back into the body to prompt growth within areas that have suffered damage. It is worth repeating that these bone marrow cells are categorically not stem cells. They are not the first in line, they aren't creators of new tissue, or even particularly special. They do, however, work well as medicinal signalling cells, so injecting them can kickstart regeneration in the affected area.

The second example of cell treatment is the use of certain human fat cells as a similar catalyst for healing and regeneration. Following exactly the same principles as BMAC treatment, we can suck out a patient's fat through liposuction, break it down into components and then inject the right cells into the body. Again, these act as medicinal signalling cells to begin the process of healing.

Fat cells science

In the realm of regenerative medicine, the potential of fat cells, or adipose tissue, is often underestimated. Moving beyond the realm of cosmetic surgery, adipose tissue presents itself as a useful player in the healing process. The key lies in micro-fragmented adipose tissue (MFAT) – a substance rich in regenerative potential that offers a new perspective on the body's innate healing abilities.

MFAT works in a similar way to BMAC – it kickstarts healing with an injection of good cells. This is because the process of breaking down fat cells isn't just a physical transformation; it's a release mechanism for potent perivascular cells known as pericytes. These pericytes, typically stationed around capillaries, are important for blood vessel formation and maintenance and leap into action in response to injury. By micro-fragmenting adipose tissue, we enhance the release of these active healing cells and create a powerful tool for regeneration.

In the spectrum of adipose tissue therapies, we encounter three distinct yet interconnected treatments: mFat, uFat and nFat. Each of these therapies processes and applies adipose-derived cells differently:

- **mFat therapy** is the simplest fat cell treatment. It involves processing adipose tissue into micro-fragments rich in pericytes and implanting it to support a broad range of regenerative treatments.

- **uFat therapy** further refines the process to create ultra-fragmented adipose tissue. This smaller fragmentation concentrates a higher number of mesenchymal cells, of the type found in bone marrow. This makes it better suited to more targeted regenerative applications.

- **nFat therapy** represents the most refined form of adipose fragmentation. Nano-fragmented adipose tissue offers a significantly enhanced surface area for interaction, making it a potent option for intensive regenerative needs.

At the heart of all fat cell regenerative power sit the pericytes. When adipose tissue is micro-, ultra- or nano-fragmented, these cells are liberated and activated. Their role is crucial. They don't just repair – they orchestrate a complex healing response involving anti-inflammatory and regenerative processes. It's a dance of cellular interplay where pericytes guide other cells towards restoration and repair. In regenerative medicine, we don't see fat cells as passive repositories of energy, but as dynamic, active agents of healing. This shift in how we understand adipose tissue opens new regenerative avenues. Why stop at just sending messages and prompts when, thanks to the latest developments in human biochemistry, we could, perhaps, control how groups of cells behave more directly?

It might help to imagine your cells working together as a sports team might. It is hard to argue against the evidence for strong captaincy. Your favourite football club is likely to be higher up the league with effective leadership on the pitch. Why wouldn't the same principle apply to human biological processes and cellular structures? You can have healthy cells that are in the right environment at the right time, but without leadership, there is no guarantee that regeneration will succeed. This is a constant frustration for those of us responsible for musculoskeletal health. Despite our best efforts, there is a degree of trial and error involved in many of our treatments. What could we achieve if we could do more than send messages and actually guide cells through regenerative tasks? With more control, we could increase the likelihood of success significantly. We could implant cells to lead, give them the materials they need and, in theory, they could do the work required.

Summary

Biology represents the most exciting frontier in regenerative medicine. New tools and techniques are developing at an ever-increasing pace. They are likely to have an impact on every level from analysing how we move to affecting us at a cellular and molecular level. It is a risk inherent in writing any book on medicine, but I strongly suspect that some of this material will be out of date by the book's publication date.

With a focus on biology, this chapter has provided a useful reminder that there is more to regenerative medicine than simply affecting how we move. The body is too much of a complex, integrated and interconnected machine for that to be the case. There is no doubt that orthopaedic surgery improves mobility, yet thanks to biology, the benefits are felt in a myriad of ways. I would argue that a hip replacement has the potential to completely change a patient's whole biology for the better. Removing chronic pain, being able to walk, getting a good night's sleep and even enjoying smiling more all have benefits at our cellular and hormonal levels. These will, in turn, have an impact on the patient's general overall health. If surgically removing and replacing a degenerated knee joint feels like a regenerative step, the knock-on effects certainly are too.

Understanding the value of regenerative medicine can only come through understanding human biological processes that operate alongside physics and chemistry. This chapter has, sadly, only been able to give you the briefest introduction to the subject through a handful of examples.

The good news is that our understanding of the biology of the body grows deeper and more complex every day. We have moved away from 'eating lots of vegetables because our parents tell us to' towards highly sophisticated treatments that combine natural biological compounds with inorganic and organic chemistry. Human technology and science have moved the goalposts and historic divisions are becoming less and less important. As lines become increasingly blurred now, one thing is for sure, there are more exciting regenerative opportunities to come.

SEVEN
The Impact Of Time

'Our time is finite' is a truism of the human condition that we ignore at great cost. We all share the same twenty-four hours a day. It is all we have. Nobody has extra. It doesn't matter who you are, how rich you are, how poor you are or how you choose to live your life; time is always a limited resource. What counts, in life, is how you spend it.

Our attitudes towards time, at least chronological time, has a big influence on how we age and the physical, chemical and biological principles we have discussed in the book's preceding chapters. It is important to carefully consider how much time you invest in regeneration and your musculoskeletal health.

We tend to think of regeneration as taking time. Without the slightest bit of professional medical input, we are happy to casually suggest resting weary joints and putting one's feet up for a while. We often say, literally, 'Time is a healer.' We instinctively know what is good for us, but we don't necessarily consider exactly how time helps us. The fact that we all experience time differently is another important factor to discuss. Our experiences of time and our health will always be unique, based on our circumstances and expectations.

Let's take a young professional sportsperson with potential to earn big money through football or basketball as an example. They might be between eighteen and twenty-five years old and consider themselves to be at the peak of their fitness and, it follows, at a prime period in their careers. For them, time is short and, should they be injured, any recovery needs to happen quickly. Given the choice between six to nine months of regenerative therapy and, say, immediate steroid injections, they might well choose the latter. Even if they understand the potential risks to their future health, time is ticking, money is at stake and speed is of the essence. After they have retired, for example, the same sports person may be happy to take their foot off the gas and invest more time in their recovery.

It is important to carefully consider your own attitude to time and regenerative medicine. How do you want to deal with any musculoskeletal issues that come up?

You will need to think about balancing short-term wins against your long-term well-being, for example:

- How much of your twenty-four hours do you need to spend working?
- How much of it do you need to be active for?
- How many hours of treatment can you fit in?
- How much time do you want to spend resting and recuperating?

Age plays a role too. You will clearly have different needs in your twenties compared to your eighties. Whatever position you find yourself in, the question is always how to make the most of the twenty-four hours a day you are given.

Physiological versus chronological time

As we get on in years, our fears around ageing are often allayed by helpful friends and family who tell us reassuringly that age is just a number. If we are looking at the calendar chronologically, this might well be true. What is the real difference between one year and the next on paper? Very little, I say.

When we talk about ageing, however, in my experience, we are rarely just talking about the passage of time. We are talking about the impact chronological time has on our bodies. We are concerned with how we feel and how effectively our physiology is working. Which bits of us are sagging? What aches and pains do we have? Is our eyesight deteriorating? Can we hear as well as we used to? This feels a different measure than mere chronology. It is something that those involved in regenerative medicine tend to define slightly differently. We might call it physiological time.

Physiological time differs from chronological time because everyone is on their own, unique path through it. You can see this in action by simply comparing different people at the same age. Let us take sixty-year-olds, for example. Some of them, a minority admittedly, are still able to show off muscular physiques in senior bodybuilding competitions. You can still see them pumping iron among a younger crowd on Miami's famous Venice Beach, for example. There are also sixty-year-old marathon runners and triathletes who compete to an incredibly impressive high standard around the world. There are other sixty-year-olds, however, with the same chronological time under their belts who struggle to climb the stairs or even walk short distances.

This is why, alongside chronological time, physiological time is such an important concept for regenerative medicine. We talk, perhaps a little unscientifically, of individual joints and organs having equivalent ages. We might describe a knee or elbow joint as being typical for a fifty-year-old. This is no doubt great to hear if you are a patient in your sixties. Less so, if you are only thirty-five. In the former, physiological time has passed slowly. In the latter case, it has passed quickly and unhealthily.

The good news is that physiological time is flexible. Our physiological ageing is influenced by a huge range of factors. In effect, all the decisions we make as we live our lives speed it up or slow it down. There is, naturally, the DNA we are born with to consider too. We will discuss illness and injury later in this chapter. The overall message, however, is that we can influence how we respond to physiological time just as we can with any other aspect of our health and well-being.

To help, it might be useful to look at an analogy from the home. How do you respond to a leaking pipe? If you ignore it, or at least delay fixing it until later, the cost of a future repair will grow. The longer you leave the problem, the worse the final outcome will be. An early fix, on the other hand, which may only cost a few pounds, avoids the issue escalating. In a similar way, treating musculoskeletal issues at the appropriate time will influence the pace at which physiological time passes for you.

Our lives are, of course, often more complex than a simple plumbing problem. A simple leak might only require a simple plastic ring to solve, after all. If we build on our initial analogy to better reflect real life, we might imagine our leak is in a luxury hotel suite.

If this is occupied at a rate of thousands of pounds a night, you might not want to disturb guests and lose out on that income to fix a minor leak. Even if you understand the risks, you might take the money today and worry about tomorrow another day. This scenario probably rings true with the way many of us view our musculoskeletal health. We are all excellent at focusing on short-term inconveniences and will typically delay facing problems because the bad news feels a long way off.

At various points in our lives, when it comes to our musculoskeletal health, we will need to make choices about what to live with, what to fix and when to fix it. We often do this having done minimal research and certainly we rarely think far enough ahead. I am suggesting, however, that we really ought to start thinking about time in more depth when considering our health. If we treated time like money, as a currency, we would achieve better outcomes. Time spent regeneratively is investing in yourself, after all. The more you do it, the better the future you can look forward to.

The right kind of exercise

Exercise is rightly seen as a great way to invest in your future physiological well-being. It is a very simple equation. Those who exercise within reason will generally have a lower physiological age than those who do not. However, not all exercise is the same.

As we discussed in the previous chapter, it is probably useful to break fitness regimes into two clear categories, Cardiovascular fitness as well as Power and Strength.

First, cardiovascular fitness keeps your heart and lungs operating in a healthy robust condition. In my experience, the vast majority of people, when they discuss exercise, refer to this category. Furthermore, many of them mean running and, specifically, they mean medium- to long-distance running. Normally, as an aside, other than elite 100 metre runners, most people only sprint at 100% when they're in peril. If you are not being chased by a tiger or escaping a fire, for example, you tend to leave some of your energy in the tank. For most normal people, fitness training means running for long periods at less than full pelt, maybe at 60–70% capacity. This is unarguably a great way to keep cardiovascularly fit. It is, of course, also why there are whole industries worth billions selling trainers, clothes, apps and training programmes built around it.

The problem with spending time on this type of exercise is that it may lower your cardiovascular age, but it can add to your musculoskeletal age. I often meet elite runners in their forties with the heart and lungs of a thirty-year-old, but the knees of someone nearer seventy. If you drill down to the details, when you run over a medium to long distance, you are repetitively moving your joints in the same direction and repeatedly lifting and dropping your body weight onto the ground. This is doubly damaging because, when you run, you run on your toes and land on a very small area of ground. It has been proven that running, compared to walking, pushes between three and five times more force up through our joints from our toes.[20] Newtonian physics, covered earlier in the book, tells us that is far from good for us. There is certainly a place for cardiovascular exercise, but an undue focus on our hearts comes back to the theme of this chapter. It is investing time in the wrong place.

I am, of course, not suggesting sitting around without doing any exercise at all. I am merely suggesting that some of the time you might currently be putting into your cardiovascular system is best redirected else-where. When you run at about 60% or 70% of your cardiovascular capacity, your muscles are not getting much beyond 50% of the workout they need. Also, the muscles receive a long, slow-burn type of workout.

The second category of fitness regimes is Power and Strength. To improve muscle performance and increase strength, we need to apply different prin-ciples that develop faster, more dynamic twitch responses. For musculoskeletal joint health, it is best to train our bodies at 80–90% of our maximum capac-ity, but unlike running, this need only be for short, intense periods. A handful of high-impact repetitions when weightlifting, for example, is way more useful to us than the 20,000 repetitions you might associate with running a long distance. This is because, in the former, the period between putting our joints under strain and recovering is shorter, which is better for promoting growth and strength. The difference becomes obvious if you compare the bodies of famous marathon runner Mo Farah and the infamous muscleman, Arnold Schwarzenegger. Elite-level rugby players who do a lot of musculoskeletal strength training can sometimes avoid surgery for major problems such as Anterior Cruciate Ligament (ACL) injuries thanks to strong muscles gained in this way.

The key message is that many of us invest a lot of our time in good cardiovascular health. Without a similar investment, however, our musculoskeletal health will lag behind.

Injury and chronic illness

Even if we plan our time meticulously, life has a way of throwing us curve balls. The time and effort we put into recovering from an unexpected injury, for example, will have a big influence on our musculoskeletal health. If you do not fix things in an appropriate timescale, you are storing up more problems for the future. A typical example is treating damaged ligaments within a knee joint. It may be possible to live with an unstable joint, but at what cost?

A patient I am aware of had a serious tear of the cruciate ligament, yet waited five years before seeking medical intervention. At the end of that period, an MRI scan showed the knee joint had been damaged beyond repair. The meniscus shock absorber had worn totally away, the cartilage was badly depleted and the bone within the joint had, through additional wear, become badly misshapen. The damage was permanent and the only course of action was a knee replacement. Delaying treatment had led to a very poor, and avoidable, outcome.

In regeneration treatment, we are rarely interested in maintaining the status quo after an injury. We can, and do, slow your physiological clock down and can, occasionally, even push it backwards. Repairing joints and structures to be stronger than they were before damage is becoming possible thanks to the cutting-edge physical, chemical and biological tools that medicine has placed at our disposal today.

As well as injury, we have to consider illness when discussing time. Musculoskeletal pain, especially if it becomes chronic, never just affects joints in isolation. Osteoarthritis in a hip joint, for example, will affect how we walk, which can, thanks to Newtonian physics, go on to affect the knees, spine, neck and shoulders. The chemistry within the body may also be altered by that painful hip, because once inflammation becomes chronic, similar symptoms are triggered across the whole body. Pain also, understandably, has a huge effect on a patient's mood, and yes, you will smile less and not sleep very well. Biologically speaking, it makes you less likely to release positive, healthy endorphins. Your body is more likely to be affected by an excess of the stress hormone, cortisol.

The current answer to long-term pain is still more often than not invasive orthopaedic surgery. Despite the fact we have described knee and hip replacements as, perhaps, overly simple mechanistic treatments elsewhere in the book, there is no question that they bring relief. By replacing a joint, and removing the cause of chronic pain, we are likely to positively affect every aspect of a patient's physics, chemistry and biology. So, while it feels odd to describe implanting a metal and plastic device as regenerative, it certainly is if we take a holistic, system-wide view of the body.

When it comes to surgery, the question I probably get asked most often is when is the right time to act. Patients understandably want to know the optimal time to have a problematic joint replaced. My initial answer is always to ask a couple of questions about pain. Are you in pain? Is that pain affecting you a lot? If the answers to both are yes, the next step is a range of diagnostic activities. We can look for arthritis or similar causes by X-ray or MRI. We can look at the physics of joint alignment, the chemical stability within the joint or any number of biological factors that may be at work. Establishing the cause of pain will make it clear if a replacement is the most appropriate treatment pathway. In my opinion, once this is done, there is no such thing as 'too early to have treatments'. Often, people wait too long for interventions out of fear. Is it safer to leave things as they are? Why risk an operation?

All the available evidence points to the fact that patients who delay are at risk of developing more severe symptoms. Importantly, this is not always in the area initially affected. If we remember the kinetic chain, a delayed hip replacement can, in a couple of years perhaps, lead to painful arthritis within the spine. Once this point has been reached, sadly, replacing the hip won't necessarily help fix both issues. A chance to alter the body's physics, chemistry and biology for the better will have been missed.

Despite the clear benefits of self-care, we do not always look after ourselves as well as we might. Life is full of distractions. If we are a parent, we tend to focus on the health of our children. Many of us spend time in our middle age managing the health of elderly relatives too. When do we have the time to look after ourselves? In terms of regenerative health, we really do need to find a way of fitting it in.

Managing our time

We all need to manage the balance between chronological and physiological time in our lives. Everybody has advice, of course, but ultimately it is down to each individual to make our own decisions and control how they age.

A good example is our attitude to the sun. On the plus side, sunbathing helps our bodies create vitamin D and can reduce our stress levels by potentially replacing cortisol with endorphins. Who doesn't enjoy lounging by the pool on holiday? A holiday is likely to be good for us, so two weeks of chronological time might have a positive result on our physiological time. That said, too much sun during your holiday might damage the collagen in your skin. In this case, too much chronological time spent by the pool will add to your physiological age. How do you handle this dilemma? How long do you sit out in the sun? Is shade more sensible?

Even in this relatively straightforward example, there are a myriad of variables to consider. Of course, there is no shortage of advice about skincare for holiday-makers. You can get guidance from your doctor or pharmacist or simply read the back of the suntan lotion bottle you've packed. The decision, however, rests with you, and most of the time, the answer is simple and logical. You already know it. Looking into the options around our joints and mobility, it soon becomes clear that things are more complex than this slightly flippant example implies.

There is so much innovation in the musculoskeletal regenerative field going on right now, it can be difficult to know where to turn. We have seen we can adopt any number of tools from across physics, chemistry and biology to slow, or even reverse, physiological time. We can refer to a joint as being seventy years old and, through treatment, make it the equivalent to forty or fifty years old. Even without specific treatment, the right exercise, correct posture, healthy eating and releasing endorphins can helpfully trim physiological time.

The thing to remember about time generally is that it doesn't stop. It doesn't wait. If you don't deal with an issue then things will move on without you. This is not something you can leave to others, either. In my experience, patients all too often leave their health in other people's hands. We might, for example, shift responsibility entirely to our GP, an alternative therapist, friends and family or even the internet. This will not necessarily help us fight the signs of musculoskeletal ageing. We need to invest time in ourselves, by ourselves, through continually asking how we feel and considering how we respond to concerns. As outlined earlier in this book, it pays to think like an engineer and spend time on research and weighing up alternatives before acting.

I'm not suggesting ignoring doctors. I am one, after all. Yet, as described above, I am very aware my patients are often bombarded with information and advice; some of it helpful, some of it less so. Even well-meaning friends and family are likely to chime in with their thoughts on what treatment is likely to work and when the best time is to have it. Everybody has a favourite anecdote about a hip or knee replacement that happened too early or too late. Sadly, it is human nature to share bad news, so you are more likely to hear about treatments that go wrong than successes. This is before we consider marketing efforts from the health, fitness and well-being industries who, of course, have their own agendas to push.

It pays for you, the patient, to spend time understanding the latest regenerative innovations. I have included some of them in the preceding chapters of this book. Many of the new tools and techniques are designed to speed up regeneration, thus saving you time. If you have a natural tendency for hesitancy, I would advise, perhaps, fighting it and moving with the times. It is worth considering a few questions:

- How aware are you of the latest medical developments?

- Is the advice that you are receiving old, traditional options out of habit?

- Do they only have the resources for certain treatments?

- Are they sticking to a choice that is perceived to be a 'safe' option?

This reluctance to embrace innovation can, in my experience, waste time. I have, if you're looking for further help, given you an insight into very powerful tools and methodologies in preceding chapters. If you are not sure, try to apply some of the regenerative principles I have shared to any suggested treatment.

Once you break it down into physics, chemistry and biology, logic and clarity will guide you.

When it comes to regenerative health and balancing chronological and physiological time, you need to make decisions for yourself based on the available evidence. There's a process you go through when you buy a house. You don't just randomly buy one because it's next door. You go to the market, you do your research, you might check local schools, and so on. You would never move house randomly, so why do that with your musculoskeletal health? There are, it seems to me, few better places to invest your time and energy.

Capturing time

Time, an elusive and finite resource, shapes our existence in profound ways. We have discussed that understanding and harnessing time is a key aspect of regenerative medicine. We haven't as yet mentioned 'capturing time' as a concept. It is something that is said about photographs, films and books. Time captured allows us to look back and access our memories. Can capturing time be applied to regenerative medicine? I'd say yes. In fact, it's a very exciting new development in the field.

Imagine your body as a masterfully crafted timepiece, a pocket watch or grandfather clock for example, with each component working in harmony. Over time, the gears may wear and its springs may weaken. It will start losing time and gradually decline in usefulness. What if, however, we had a detailed blueprint of this timepiece in its prime? A map that could guide us in repairing and realigning each component to its original state. We could keep our timepiece going forever.

Today, we can capture our biological and biomechanical data in more detail than ever. We can make a blueprint of ourselves, our gears and our springs. In theory, with the advent of digital technology, we now have the means to store a comprehensive digital record of our physical selves, our own 'Digital Body Bank'. This repository, comprising X-rays, MRI and CT scans, could serve as a timeless reference to our optimal physiological state. Furthermore, AI-enhanced motion capture technologies like MAI-Motion extend this capability to capture our movement and biomechanics in a digital format.

Consider this a similar experience to capturing a photograph at a moment when we look and feel our best. Just as we cherish a photo taken at a joyful, peak moment in our lives, storing our 'Digital Body Bank' becomes a pivotal step in our health journey. It's a snapshot of our physiological prime and a benchmark for future regeneration efforts.

Such a body bank becomes a tool of immense value. In times of need, it could become our guide and blueprint, enabling medical professionals to reconstruct and rejuvenate bodies with precision. Capturing time in this way is more than just preservation – it's an act of foresight and empowerment. It might not technically be time travel, but it is certainly a superhuman response to the problems of getting older.

Summary

Managing your musculoskeletal health is always a good use of your time. It can, admittedly, feel difficult to think of the future because life is full of immediate distractions, but the effort will undoubtedly pay off in the long run. Do it well and physiological time will run behind chronological time for you. We have all seen people who surprise us by looking, and perhaps acting, younger than we might expect them to be. This is the theory in action. It is perfectly achievable to have a musculoskeletal system that is younger than it ought to be if you measure it in physiological time rather than in chronological time. This is because, by applying regenerative principles, you can slow physiological time and, in the case of treating injury or disease, even sometimes reverse it.

As a doctor practising regenerative medicine, I particularly enjoy telling patients they have the joints of a younger person. It is less fun to tell someone their hip or knee joint, for example, is physiologically ten years older than they are. Achieving the former, rather than the latter, comes from treating time seriously. It is difficult, as we all lead increasingly busy lives, but we must make time for our bones, joints and muscles. We all have the same twenty-four hours a day to manage. How will you spend yours?

Investing time, that most precious of commodities, into your musculoskeletal system means doing the right exercise and choosing the right treatments for damage or illness. Acting sooner rather than later will always pay off in the long run. Time is a currency I would encourage you to use wisely and capture while you can.

EIGHT

Regenerating Like A Superhuman

A s we reach the final chapter, I think it is worth revisiting the reason I chose to write *Regeneration By Design* in the first place. Unusually for an orthopaedic surgeon and an engineer, I can summarise my position as wanting to keep patients away from my operating table. My regenerative principles are designed to make sure you keep healthy and mobile as you age, with minimal intervention. To achieve this, I am aware I need to do more than share theory, so let's practice the 'Six Superhuman Steps'. I need to give you everyday, practical tips to protect your musculoskeletal health. I need to help you live a regenerative life like a real life, honest-to-goodness superhuman.

Before I start, it's worth pausing to reflect on life itself. We owe our existence to an incredibly complex network of interconnected physical, chemical and biological systems and processes. Any breakdown in this network leads to degeneration in our health. It is not overdramatic to say that major breakdowns tend to put our lives at risk. To prevent this, a healthy body, like all living things, self-regulates and balances degeneration and regeneration. All living organisms are on a constant quest for homeostasis: a state of natural stability. This balance becomes harder to maintain as we age and I have discussed the challenges this presents in previous chapters. Problem-solving in this context is far from easy. Understanding the component parts of our body is one thing, but living regeneratively requires a shift in perspective. We constantly need to zoom out and take a system-wide view.

The practical suggestions I make in this chapter are the result of a lot of hard systematic thinking. This is different from the rather mechanistic thinking sometimes associated with medical treatments. Simply saying a problem can be fixed with a single isolated intervention feels like an oversimplification, for example. This is something to bear in mind if you ever have an appointment with a doctor.

In thinking systematically, I have tried not to rely on old familiar medical dogma. Rather than solely thinking like a doctor, I have, at every turn, tried to think like an engineer too. I have gone back to first principles and applied science to the problem of how to live like a superhuman. This has led to a six-step plan.

I made it clear in my introduction that this wasn't a self-help book and I am not a guru, so this might be a surprise. However, you can relax, my six steps are not rules. They are simply things that might be useful for you to consider as you begin to apply some of the concepts I've raised in *Regeneration By Design* to your life.

SIX SUPERHUMAN STEPS – M³D³ FORMULA

1. Minimise disturbance

To set the stage for effective regeneration, it is essential to first remove any aggravating external factors. For instance, addressing a knee problem can't be fully effective if a separate issue (eg, a stone in your shoe) is still impacting your walking pattern.

2. Modify chemistry

After external disturbances are addressed and physics is corrected, the focus shifts to the body's chemical balance. Ensuring that the molecular composition of joints, muscles, bones and tissues is conducive to regeneration is crucial.

3. Maximise biological benefits

Concurrently with chemistry, optimising the body's biological processes is key to fostering growth and regeneration. This includes everything from emotional well-being (such as the benefits of smiling) to physiological aspects like sleep, circulation, hormone levels and vitamin intake.

4. Determine the physics

Poor posture, misaligned joints and unhealthy movement patterns directly contribute to musculoskeletal degeneration, as explained by Newtonian physics. Incorporating elements of physics such as light, magnetism, sound waves and energy can play a significant role in correcting these issues. (See MAI Motion in the Further Reading.)

5. Digital body banking (Digital Twin)

In this crucial step, we embrace the concept of a 'Digital Body Bank', also known as the Digital Twin. By digitally capturing and storing comprehensive records of our physiological health and biomechanics, including X-rays, MRI, CT scans and MAI-Motion data, we create a digital blueprint of our optimal state. This repository serves as a vital reference for guiding future regeneration efforts, ensuring that we have a clear benchmark to return to in case of injury or age-related changes.

6. Decisions

Time influences every aspect of the regeneration process. Delays or periods of inaction often lead to suboptimal outcomes. This step involves making informed decisions about the timing of treatments and balancing immediate needs against long-term health and well-being.

$$R = \sum_{n=1}^{\infty} n\, M^3 D^3$$

The regeneration formula

By following these six steps, individuals can approach their regenerative health journey in a comprehensive, scientifically grounded manner, aligning physical, chemical, biological and temporal factors for optimal health outcomes.

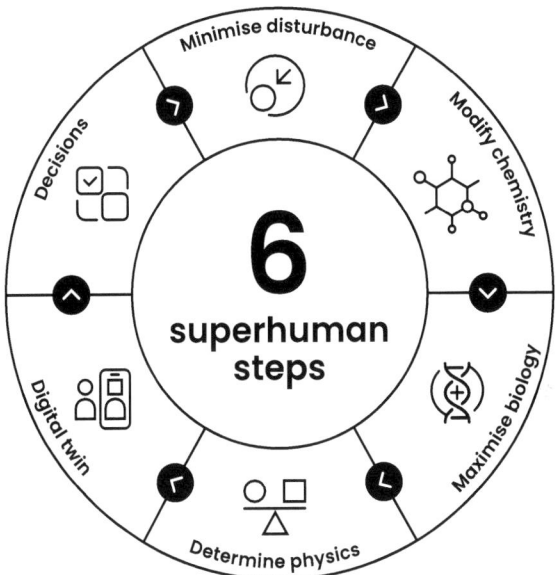

As an orthopaedic surgeon working in regenerative medicine, I spend my time constantly checking how I influence each of the six areas outlined above. As regeneration is an ongoing process, it is likely that the six steps will operate as a cycle. If you want to regenerate like a superhuman, however, considering each step separately is a good place to start.

Moving like a superhuman

How do you apply the six steps into your life? Let's start at number one. The reference to having a stone in one's shoe may be slightly flippant but, as we discussed briefly in the chapter on Newtonian physics, a poor choice of footwear is a good example of a physical factor that can aggravate degeneration. One thinks of high fashion and the pain associated with wearing inappropriate high heels, but even a worn-out sole or worn-down heel can prove problematic. It is always worth investing in high-quality shoes and replacing them regularly. I know you are very likely to have an old favourite pair of shoes that you love despite the fact they are falling apart. Sad to say, it is time to say goodbye as they might not be doing you any good. The same is especially true of running shoes. I would always recommend athletes get themselves a fitting from a specialist supplier before investing in a pair to hit the road in.

The way we lift and carry items with weight to them can also form aggravating musculoskeletal disturbances. We are all probably aware that lifting and carrying heavy items risks injury thanks to the manual handling education associated with workplace health and safety training. It is rarely a thrillingly exciting subject, but does need to be taken seriously. We should also consider what we carry outside of work. Shoulder bags slung over one shoulder or across our bodies, for example, can quickly become problematic as they get bigger and heavier. This is especially true if we, as many of us do, carry laptops and tablets around with us. A useful, if slightly imprecise, rule of thumb is the weight of a shoulder bag should never exceed 10% of your body weight.

Talking of technology, where is your monitor when you work at your PC? Is your eyeline correct? Is your desk at the right height? Is your keyboard the right distance from your body? Does your mouse support your wrists? Does your chair support your back? Details such as these, small and incidental as they might seem, represent the first steps on the journey to living regeneratively.

It all comes back to Newtonian physics. It doesn't matter how many other treatments you consider, which drugs you are prescribed or which supplements you take, if you carry a bag that's too heavy on your shoulder every day, you are going to be lopsided and your spine will not be able to regenerate healthily.

Even if you align all the physical aspects of your life with regenerative principles perfectly, normal everyday activities will still cause your muscles and joints to degenerate. Standing all day, walking long distances or light exercise will still, more than likely, need a period of recovery. It has become common for sportspeople to aid similar musculoskeletal recovery through the use of ice baths. The science of this is generally sound and, in summary, involves shocking the body's cells into regenerative behaviour. Once the ice effect is removed, blood flow is increased and cells are more likely to regenerate. Is this something you can adopt as an individual? It might be worth trying. Running the cold tap rather than the hot tap for a quick bath after exercise is possibly helpful. There are, of course, heavily marketed specific products making claims for 'cryo-treatment' or 'cryo-therapy'. The evidence of their effectiveness, however, is probably best described as questionable.

Another common regenerative practice adopted by elite sportspeople is oxygen-based. Training in hyperbaric oxygen chambers, for example, or at high altitude locations with thin air, is an effective way of increasing the rate and efficiency of the body's processing of oxygen. On the understanding that few of us are likely to move to the Himalayas and train, there are a range of 'exercise with (and without) oxygen' products and treatments available to individuals. As with ice baths, the benefits they bring to everyday regeneration, as opposed to Olympic-level athletes, are difficult to prove.

The message we can take away from the above, however, is the importance of our breathing. The circulation of healthy oxygenated blood cells is, after all, a key ingredient in regeneration. The way our blood gets oxygenated is by passing over alveoli, small balloon-shaped structures, in our lungs. Our alveoli provide the equivalent of almost two tennis courts of surface area in each of us. This means we can process up to 6 litres of air with each breath. It is possibly a surprising fact, then, that we normally use just 20% of our lung capacity. We don't routinely replace all the stale air and carbon dioxide in our lungs with fresh, oxygen-rich air. Regularly practising deep breathing, as you might in a yoga class, for example, is a great regenerative tool.

I share the above to prompt thought rather than act as specific recommendations. My main message is to put some thought into your physical activities. Are they aligned with regenerative principles? The answers might help you decide if you need to carry your laptop everywhere with you. You might buy an alternative kneeling office stool or even decide to work standing up more often. You might get around to throwing away your old favourite shoes and investing in new quality footwear too. There are countless other examples. What is important is the removal of physical factors that disturb the equilibrium of your musculoskeletal system and their replacement with healthier alternatives.

As one final note on small physical changes you can make to your routine, I am forced to suggest something I know many readers will find slightly controversial. Imagine being faced with a choice between a lift and the stairs. I don't mind what you picture exactly, but you have to decide between the exertion of climbing, say, a couple of flights of stairs or pressing a button and being whisked upstairs without any effort at all. Thinking about your health, which is it?

I know this may come as a surprise, but I am going to suggest, in this scenario, ignoring the stairs and jumping straight in the lift. The reason we believe stairs are best is because, in the UK particularly, we seem to value cardiovascular health above musculoskeletal health. A raised heartbeat, even for five minutes as we tackle a few steps, is prized above the well-being of our joints. As I explained in the chapter on physics in *Regeneration By Design,* we put huge additional forces through our knees when we run. The same is true when we fight gravity to go up and down stairs. The latter is worse for our joints as we are generally moving more quickly and our feet land more heavily as we descend.

It is worth reiterating that I am not suggesting cardiovascular exercise is in any way inherently bad for you or you should do less of it. I am just suggesting it needs careful thought, because not all activity supports regeneration. I would say, given the choice, a regular weekend hike or cycle ride in the countryside, for example, is a much more sensible way of getting cardiovascular exercise than running up and down stairs occasionally.

Eating like a superhuman

As well as how we move, what and how we eat has a significant impact on our regenerative health. The familiar adage, 'You are what you eat', is true in the sense that the biology and chemistry of our bodies are certainly affected by what we ingest and how we ingest it.

The world is full of advice on diets, some of it good, medically speaking, and some of it less so, but I do not intend to go into general diet advice here. There are literally millions of other books available for that. Whatever model their authors use to describe the ideal diet, the objective and output are almost always the same: the balance of what we eat – protein, carbohydrate and fats – influences how we live. In general, if we eat wisely, we will live well. Little advice, however, is specifically about musculoskeletal health. Even less is about a superhuman response, so I am going to focus on that.

Vitamins, as we have discussed alongside biology earlier in the book, are incredibly useful regeneratively. Picturing Regency-period sailors suffering from scurvy with no teeth, bleeding gums and failing limbs provides a reminder of the value of vitamin C. It is vital to the production of the collagen that literally holds us together. We also discussed the importance of vitamin D and its role in the production of calcium and our bone health, vitamin E and its benefits for our skin, the impact of vitamin A on our eyesight and vitamin B's role in supporting our neurovascular network and, apparently, fighting male pattern baldness.

The list of good healthy things to eat is long and varied. The question, in a regenerative life, is how much of them you can get from your normal diet and what, if any, additional supplements you should take. Most of us, without a degenerative problem, should not need to take supplements as part of a normal diet. Following advice and sticking to five portions of fruit and vegetables a day, for example, should be fine. Supplements can, however, be a useful addition to your normal diet in certain circumstances. It is important to follow the manufacturer's guidelines at all times and seek professional advice with any concerns. It is also worth noting that the diet and nutrition industry is rife with pseudo-doctors and self-appointed advisors with questionable qualifications. I am, ultimately, saying it pays to be selective about who you listen to.

It is, of course, not unusual for elite athletes to supplement their diets. Before a marathon, for example, an elite runner will take on additional carbohydrates, knowing they are about to burn a lot of energy. Weightlifters will supplement their diets with extra protein in the runup to a competition because extra muscle mass might give them a competitive advantage. It is common for most elite sports teams to call on the services of nutritionists to help with such work these days.

In the same way, a patient undergoing musculoskeletal regenerative treatment might need to top up their biochemistry with appropriate supplements. This is especially true before and after surgery.

Superhuman regeneration and your doctor

Although I am aware this is a sweeping generalisation, it seems the British attitude to regenerative problems is typically to adopt a stiff upper lip and simply move on. One of the frustrations of treating musculoskeletal problems is the fact that many patients avoid treatment, preferring to *carry on regardless*. I am not sure if this is caused by a desire to be courageous or an inherent fear of hearing the truth. In reality, the complexity of human psychology means it is probably a combination of the two. Whatever the cause, it certainly counts as an unhelpful attitude. It should not come as a surprise to hear I think it is definitely not part of living a regenerative life, either. 'Pushing through' pain, ignoring discomfort and delaying seeking professional advice will, in my experience, always make problems worse.

It may be impractical, of course, to visit the doctor with every single twinge, slight ache or instance of pain. A general rule of thumb is to get professional advice if any single instance of musculoskeletal pain lasts for over forty-eight hours. Then, seeking further investigation is probably wise. It is typical NHS protocol to start by visiting your GP. It is, however, worth doing a little research first. Just because somebody is local to you does not mean they are best placed to advise on musculoskeletal issues. You can always ask your GP to refer you to a specific specialist or clinic.

Whoever undertakes it, this further investigation will vary. It is common, however, for patients to request an X-ray. The general perception of X-rays as a strong diagnostic tool is, however, often misplaced. X-rays are very good at identifying bone fractures, but of limited use beyond that. This is important, because I would estimate that 99% of cases of musculoskeletal pain are caused by soft tissue injuries. If you have pain but can put weight on a joint, it is extremely unlikely that anything is broken. This makes an X-ray pointless. This doesn't, however, stop doctors occasionally using them to placate and reassure worried patients.

Magnetic Resonance Imaging (MRI) scans are required to diagnose problems with soft tissues. They can be difficult to arrange on the NHS, but they are becoming more available through private medicine. The issue with MRI scans is they are dependent on an individual doctor or radiologist's interpretation. Different specialists can look at an MRI scan and see slightly different things. If you are arranging an MRI scan, it is useful to assess the skills and experience of the supervising medical professional. Simply taking the scan is only part of the role. Writing an accurate report is, if anything, the more important task. As an orthopaedic surgeon I often see MRI reports and, before making a judgement, I check the reputation and seniority of the author. This, in fact, applies to any feature of regenerative treatment. It can prove a mistake to simply follow guidance from a place of dogmatic trust in doctors.

You are the expert in your own body and it pays to invest time in understanding your health and well-being. Why wouldn't you take a detailed interest? Your regenerative health is vitally important. It is worth arming yourself with as much knowledge as you can to avoid the need to follow any advice from a position of blind trust.

By looking after yourself, and living a regenerative life through the physical and diet steps outlined above, my hope is that you would avoid any form of surgery. This goes back to the reason for writing *Regeneration By Design*: to keep you away from the operating table. Despite our best efforts, however, sometimes an operation cannot be avoided. If that's the case, I recommend you choose your surgeon carefully and approach any treatment as a joint effort. It's vital you understand every detail of the proposed procedure and feel comfortable proceeding. The discussion should be as long and in as much depth as you need. A good surgeon will take the time to make sure your consent is from a fully informed position.

One idea that is useful to bear in mind is that the first surgery is always the best chance to fix an issue; the first bite of the cherry is the sweetest. If repeated surgery is recommended, it is worth asking why and, perhaps, trying to look for an alternative. Again, a good surgeon will help you work out the right procedure for your circumstances.

My point, overall, is to take professional advice with a pinch of salt. It is important to always assess who is giving it to you, and why. Applying the four pillars of my regeneration principles – physics, chemistry, biology and time – will help too.

This approach is, however, not just about healing from injuries or surgeries; it's about a proactive lifestyle that consistently aligns with the principles of regenerative living. This might mean incorporating physics into your daily routine, for example, by being mindful of your posture, your movements and your physical environment. Why not choose ergonomically designed furniture or opt for footwear that supports your natural gait? Why not check if your balanced diet includes essential nutrients that support cellular regeneration?

Are you getting adequate sleep, managing stress effectively and maintaining hormonal balance? Would a digital record of your optimal health help you make more informed medical decisions? What about timing? When is the right moment for a surgical procedure or starting a new exercise regimen? Finding answers to these, and countless questions like them, based on a sound understanding of science, engineering and design is my definition of superhuman living.

Considering the above, we can see that regenerating like a superhuman involves more than just following a set of steps. It requires a mindset shift. It's about making conscious choices every day that are in harmony with the principles of regenerative living. It means being an active participant in your health care, understanding the why and how of each recommendation, and ensuring that every aspect of your lifestyle supports your regenerative goals.

By adopting this comprehensive approach, you not only heal and protect your body, but also enhance your overall well-being, staying true to the concept of *Regeneration By Design*. This way of living empowers you to take control of your health, leading to a more resilient, regenerated self.

Summary

If we return to the beginning of this chapter, living a regenerative life means considering six steps: minimising disturbance, correcting the physics, maintaining the correct chemistry, maximising biological benefits, re-integrating motion and considering the context of time.

This structure is the closest I get in this book to the kind of handy mnemonic that you might expect in a self-help guide book. I am very aware, though, that you are all individuals with unique musculoskeletal systems. You will, no doubt, find certain of my ideas chime with you and others do not. It's important that you pick and choose advice that fits with you and your lifestyle. The same is true when it comes to the exercise and diet guidance in this chapter. You might find vitamin supplements helpful and take the occasional ice bath. Again, if it helps you, I consider this a success.

My final thought on living a regenerative life is that doctors and medical professionals are there to provide help and advice but you should, at all times, be in a position where you can make educated decisions about your musculoskeletal health. My wish is that you feel empowered to take action rather than follow doctors blindly out of habit. I want you to feel in control. That is the ultimate superhuman lesson I can give you: *you are in full control of your own health.*

Remember the regeneration formula and think like a superhuman.

$$R = \sum_{n=1}^{\infty} n\, M^3 D^3$$

Conclusion

As I draw *Regeneration By Design* to a close, it is worth reflecting on why I wanted to write the book in the first place. Frustrated by how I see today's patients handle ageing, I set a goal of encouraging readers to consider musculoskeletal health and regenerative medicine anew. In doing so, I wanted them to enjoy a plan for a future that didn't include troubling my operating theatre for joint replacement surgery. I also wanted to share an up-to-date view of regenerative tools and techniques that challenged some of the behind-the-times dogmatic thinking I still see in modern medicine. I certainly hoped, as I put pen to paper, to move the debate onward from dated textbooks towards current, evidence-based innovations. Regenerative science has made huge steps forward in recent years thanks, in large part, to sports medicine. This is something I definitely wanted to celebrate too.

Today, we have the knowledge and the power to understand more about regenerative processes than ever. Regenerative medicine has become an exciting and ever-evolving space in which to work. It is undoubtedly continuing to develop as I write. Who knows? It may be that some of the science included may already have been superseded by cleverer ideas before this book is published. If this is the case, I apologise, but encourage you to throw yourself into researching the latest developments for yourself.

We have landed on a key message of the book. We currently do not spend enough time looking after ourselves. I hope that once they have read *Regeneration By Design*, readers will see the value of investing time in the design work required to have healthy ageing planned. Surely, it is too important a thing to leave to chance.

To help plan for a regenerative future, I have shared scientific principles from across physics, chemistry and biology. We all probably remember science lessons from school. If your memories are like mine, learning mass and force equations, watching coloured flames in a Bunsen burner and memorising the component parts of leaves and tree roots probably did not feel hugely applicable to your life. I hope I have been able to present regenerative science differently. If

I have done my job correctly, you will know why the principles in this book are important and how they will help you age well. I have discussed the importance of time in regenerative health too. This, together with the three sciences, adds up to the four core principles that have made up the bulk of *Regeneration By Design*'s content.

We all know that prevention is better than cure, but we will inevitably get injured or sick during our lives. The superhuman approach to healing is to design our recovery and to use the regeneration principle to beat time and degeneration. We instinctively know acting promptly is better than leaving things too late. In writing *Regeneration By Design,* I have taken time to reflect on what these things mean. How should we manage our musculoskeletal system as we age? Some of my conclusions seem ridiculously straightforward. You can avoid back pain as you age by keeping hydrated in your youth, for example. Other issues are more complex. Your cells' interconnectivity begins to fall apart when the collagen in your joints degenerates. All my recommendations are very much based on sound, proven science. I've been lucky that throughout my career I've been able to draw on both high-end clinical practice and academic research.

As well as science, the book has asked some philosophical questions. What is life? What does ageing well mean? What is 'superhuman'? What is a healthy balance between regeneration and degeneration? We discussed the body's natural equilibrium, known as homeostasis, which is a critical concept in regenerative health. We are, as living organisms, destined to degenerate. The fact we all die in the end is a universal and unavoidable truth. We can, however, slow the process and make our journey as smooth and painless as possible.

Having established we have a finite amount of time on the planet, it is perhaps understandable if you have, as a reader, flicked straight to the conclusion. If you have, relax. I'll summarise my key advice for you.

It is important that, before you consider regenerative changes to your life, you minimise disruption. If there is a splinter from your tennis racket handle working its way into your hand, for example, you need to fix that before fixing your serve. The next step is to correct how we move in terms of Newtonian physics. This might include the bracing, strapping or taping of joints. Chemistry comes next. This can be used to create a stable environment for cells to regenerate in. Talking of regenerative cells, we can affect the body's biological processes too. Time is also a factor in all regeneration processes. Knowing when, and how, to get treatment is as important as choosing the treatment itself.

It is, of course, likely that you'll need professional advice at some point in your regenerative planning. This brings me to the main reason *Regeneration By*

Design exists. Once you have read the book, I hope you will feel inspired to plan how you age for *yourself*. It doesn't matter how many men and women in white coats you see, how much experience they have or what certificates they have on their walls. It pays to be cynical and do your own regenerative research. *Regeneration By Design* is my contribution to the cause. It aims to provide a dispassionate, logical view of how regenerative medicine might help you age. Logic is part of what makes us different from animals, after all. We can look at the evidence and make our own decisions. We don't have to give up control to anyone else.

I have talked about engineering principles throughout the book, but perhaps it is worth mentioning architecture too. You do not generally buy a house off the shelf. You definitely don't let an architect make all the decisions for you. That would feel incredibly risky. Instead, you need to take the time to explain the house of your dreams. It helps to understand a little of the science behind house construction as you do, so you can articulate what you want in terms your architect will understand.

I hope *Regeneration By Design* will help you discuss your regenerative health with a similar sense of partnership with medical professionals. You are planning your future in exactly the same way you might when you chat with an architect. The only difference is that you are discussing your body, rather than your home or office. We are designing superhumans, after all.

It is an ongoing process though, because things never run smoothly as we get older. The old cliche about the only constant being change applies to regeneration. I perhaps ought to have called the book *Regeneration By Design and Redesign and Redesign and Redesign, ad infinitum.* Being too fixed in your ways isn't helpful.

If you have read this far, I think you have everything you need to design a regenerative future. There is nothing that says musculoskeletal pain and discomfort are inevitable. There is no reason to expect joint replacement surgery in your old age. The decisions you will make today and tomorrow will help you avoid them both and power you towards a superhuman life. It is worth reiterating the point I made thirty-odd thousand words ago. Despite being an orthopaedic surgeon, I do not want to see you in my operating theatre any time soon.

I shall leave you by wishing you a long, happy and mobile regenerative life.

Further Reading

Motion Artificial Intelligence – MAI Motion

M AI stands for 'Motion Artificial Intelligence' and it's a term you will soon hear a lot about in musculoskeletal circles. It is the first time that technology has become available through which we can both understand human movement and interlink it from one joint to another. It is exciting because, prior to MAI, we have tended to focus on one joint at a time. Our ambitions have been limited by the limitations of MRIs, CT scans and X-rays. When we look at them, they're only two-dimensional. CT and MRI scans are static too.

Nowadays, the technology is here to make previous limitations meaningless. We have the computer processing power and digital memory available to look at all of our joints at the same time, in three dimensions and in motion. We're very close to joining everything together. Imagine having a view of all our body movement: studying how your shoulder joint affects your hip joint and your hip joint affects your knee joint, for example, all in the same sitting. We now have the technology to look at a whole body's movement at one go. Over the last ten years, we have achieved something called a 'Digital Kinematic Signature'. This means we can see the way you move when you are healthy. Spotting changes can predict and diagnose disease or injury. This technology is available now. For a Digital Kinematic Signature, we can use a video recorded through a mobile phone camera.

Having a simple video removes the subjectivity from assessing the musculoskeletal system. You may visit an orthopaedic surgeon or a chiropractor. They say that the way you squat is 'funny' or that your knee is going a bit too far one way or not far enough in another. It's not exactly an exact science. With video and modern computing power, we can quantify all this movement. The computer can give you a number that is reliable every time. This is a fundamental breakthrough. This is where the artificial intelligence in Motion Artificial Intelligence comes into its own with deep learning and computer vision. By comparing millions of data sets, Motion Artificial Intelligence provides a diagnostic tool more objective and powerful than any doctor, however skilled, could ever hope to be. Better yet, it is available on your mobile phone.

Motion Artificial Intelligence can now monitor and define the physics of movement physics for you. There may be a time, no doubt sooner than we might imagine, when recording your movement will become part of your everyday routine and changes flagged and diagnosed automatically by AI. By storing this data, we can capture time too. We can link physics and time together with Motion Artificial Intelligence which, we know, is fundamental in regeneration.

You can find our more at https://maimotion.com.

Notes

1   Letter to Robert Hooke, 5 February 1676, in HW
Turnbull (ed). Correspondence of Isaac Newton
vol 1 (1959), https://libquotes.com/isaac-
newton/quotes/giants, accessed 12 February
2024

2   Ferreira ML, 'Global, regional, and national
burden of low back pain, 1990–2020, its
attributable risk factors, and projections to
2050: A systematic analysis of Global Burden
of Disease Study 2021', *The Lancet* (June 2023),
https://doi.org/10.1016/S2665-9913(23)00098-X,
accessed 10 April 2024

3   Cancer Research UK, www.cancerresearchuk.
org/health-professional/cancer-statistics/
statistics-by-cancer-type/lung-cancer/risk-
factors, accessed 24 February 2024

4   Yeomans C, Kenny IC, Cahalan R, et al, 'The
    Incidence of Injury in Amateur Male Rugby
    Union: A Systematic Review and Meta-
    Analysis', *Sports Medicine*, 2018;48(4):837–
    848, www.ncbi.nlm.nih.gov/pmc/articles/
    PMC5856893, accessed 10 April 2024
5   Snowden DJ, and Boone ME, 'A Leader's
    Framework for Decision Making', *Harvard
    Business Review* (November 2007), https://hbr.
    org/2007/11/a-leaders-framework-for-decision-
    making, accessed
    10 April 2024
6   Caplan AI, 'Mesenchymal stem cells', *Journal
    of Orthopaedic Research*, 1991; 9: 641–650,
    https://onlinelibrary.wiley.com/doi/10.1002/
    jor.1100090504, accessed 24 February 2024
7   Caplan AI, 'Mesenchymal Stem Cells: Time
    to Change the Name!' *Stem Cells Translational
    Medicine*, 2017, 6: 1445–1451, https://doi.
    org/10.1002/sctm.17-0051
8   Lister J, 'On the Antiseptic Principle in the
    Practice of Surgery', *The British Medical Journal*
    (September 1867), www.ncbi.nlm.nih.gov/pmc/
    articles/PMC2310614, accessed 10 April 2024
9   Ataman AD, Vatanoğlu-Lutz EE, Yıldırım G,
    'Medicine in stamps–Ignaz Semmelweis and
    Puerperal Fever', *Journal of the Turkish-German
    Gynecological Association* (March 2013), https://
    pubmed.ncbi.nlm.nih.gov/24592068, accessed
    10 April 2024

10 Loeser RF, Goldring SR, Scanzello CR, Goldring MB, 'Osteoarthritis: A disease of the joint as an organ', *Arthritis & Rheumatology*, 2012;64(6):1697–1707, https://pubmed.ncbi.nlm.nih.gov/22392533, accessed 10 April 2024

11 National Science Foundation, 'Gravitational waves from colossal black holes found using "cosmic clocks"', ScienceDaily (29 June 2023), www.sciencedaily.com/releases/2023/06/230629125650.htm, accessed 10 April 2024

12 Glenn Research Center, 'Newton's Laws Of Motion', NASA (no date), www1.grc.nasa.gov/beginners-guide-to-aeronautics/newtons-laws-of-motion, accessed 10 April 2024

13 One Newton is defined as the force required to accelerate one kilogram at the rate of one metre per second, every second.

14 Buchbinder R, Green S, Youd JM, 'Corticosteroid injections for shoulder pain', *Cochrane Database of Systematic Reviews 2003*, Issue 1. Art. No: CD004016, https://pubmed.ncbi.nlm.nih.gov/12535501, accessed 25 February 2024

15 Kraft TL, & Pressman SD, 'Grin and Bear It: The Influence of Manipulated Facial Expression on the Stress Response', *Psychological Science*, (2012) 23(11), 1372–1378, https://doi.org/10.1177/0956797612445312, accessed 24 February 2024

16 ibid

17 Fitriana V, Santoso A & Dharmana E, 'The
   Experiences and Meanings of Nurses' Smiles to
   Patients in the Emergency Department', *Nurse
   Media Journal of Nursing* (2020) 11(1),
   104–113, https://doi.org/10.14710/nmjn.
   v11i1.28377, accessed
   24 February 2024

18 Han G, et al, 'Refractive Corneal Inlay
   for Presbyopia in Emmetropic Patients in
   Asia: 6-Month Clinical Outcomes', *BMC
   Ophthalmology* (2019) 19(1), https://doi.
   org/10.1186/s12886-019-1069-2, accessed 24
   February 2024

19 Zarif MJ, Alió JL, Barrio JL, Miguel MP,
   Jawad K, & Makdissy N, 'Corneal Stromal
   Regeneration: A Review of Human Clinical
   Studies in Keratoconus Treatment', *Frontiers
   in Medicine* (2021) 8, https://doi.org/10.3389/
   fmed.2021.650724, accessed 24 February 2024

20 Swain DP, et al, 'Impact Forces of Walking and
   Running at the Same Intensity', *The Journal
   of Strength & Conditioning Research* (April
   2016) 30(4), https://pubmed.ncbi.nlm.nih.
   gov/27003452, accessed 16 April 2024

Acknowledgements

First and foremost, I extend my deepest gratitude to my parents and my brother, whose nurturing and guidance have been the bedrock of my personal and professional life. Their wisdom and unconditional love have provided me with the strength and resilience to pursue my aspirations in becoming a medical doctor. Their examples have taught me the value of dedication and hard work, qualities that have been essential throughout the writing of this book.

I am equally indebted to my family – my steadfast wife, Bethan, and our wonderful children, Morgan, Ffion and Owen. Their boundless support and engagement with my sometimes endless discussions about systematic thinking and the beauty of regenerative medicine, even during our Christmas gatherings, have been nothing short of miraculous. Their patience and critical engagement with my ideas have been instrumental in helping me discover the regenerative equation for our lives, reinforcing my belief that the only limits that exist are those we impose on ourselves.

Special thanks to Professors James Richardson and Len Nokes, whose mentorship in the fundamentals of regenerative medicine and the integration of engineering principles, respectively, have profoundly shaped my approach to this field. Their insights have been pivotal in laying the groundwork for the concepts presented in *Regeneration By Design*.

My gratitude extends to Kar Hao Teoh, a close friend and master architect of regenerative pathways that propel medicine to new heights. The work of my mentor, Amit Chandratreya, has deepened my understanding of the logic behind our surgical practices, continually pushing the boundaries of orthopaedic surgery and regenerative medicine.

I must also thank Ruth Virgo for her friendship and dynamic energy. Her ability to translate and implement my ideas has been instrumental in rediscovering my own potential. Her unwavering belief in my capabilities and her encouragement have been crucial in pushing me to explore further and complete this book.

Special thanks to my friend, 'Maha', Mr K Mahalingam, and Malcolm Pearson, whose philosophy that 'we are not here for a long time, we are here for a good time,' echoes through the pursuit of regenerative medicine.

My appreciation extends to my friends at Harley Street, London – Simon Marsh and Clair Linnane – for enduring my relentless stream of ideas and continually encouraging me to test the boundaries within regenerative medicine.

I am also thankful for the vibrant academic communities at the University of Lincoln, including the departments of Sport, Biomedical Science and Computer Vision, whose support has enriched my research and development.

Lastly, my family, friends, mentors and trainers in Wales deserve a profound acknowledgement; your guidance in medical, scientific and engineering training has been pivotal in my journey. Thank you all for guiding me through the evolving landscape of regenerative medicine.

The Author

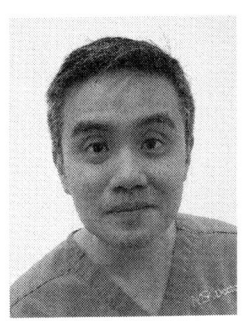

Professor Paul YF Lee, MB BCh, MFSEM (UK), MSc (Sports Med), PhD, FEBOT, FRCS (Tr & Orth) stands at the forefront of regenerative medicine, skilfully blending his orthopaedic surgical expertise with innovative engineering insights. His career began with a deep interest in the complexities of arthritis and sports injuries, propelling him towards an MSc in Sports Medicine and a PhD in Medical Engineering and setting the foundation for his impactful journey in medicine.

Authoring over eighty clinical publications, Professor Lee has markedly influenced regenerative therapy, especially in enhancing recovery processes for elite athletes. His work in developing advanced treatments such as mFat, STARR-ACL, SPAIRE, Bikini hip, TWISTKR, A-PRP, and cell therapies for osteoarthritis has redefined therapeutic standards. His introduction of innovative injection protocols broadens the spectrum of advanced regenerative treatments available, both surgical and non-surgical.

Professor Lee's role extends beyond clinical practice. He is a pioneer in applying AI and machine learning in the MSK Computer Vision Lab, revolutionising human kinematics with his invention of MAI-Motion technology. This groundbreaking work underscores the productive convergence of medical science and engineering, propelling the discipline of regenerative medicine forward.

Professor Lee regularly treats patients at the Regenerative Clinic, the London Cartilage Clinic and the Gilmore's Groin team at the London Sports Injury Clinic. Over the years, he has built up a network to exchange knowledge with an international team of surgeons to remain at the cutting edge of innovation.

Find out more:

⊕ regenman.com

Printed in Great Britain
by Amazon

52217369R00115